The
Food
Intolerance
Handbook

Sharla Race

The Food Intolerance Handbook:
Your Guide to Understanding Food Intolerance, Food
Sensitivities, Food Chemicals, and Food Allergies

Published 2017
ISBN: 9781907119606

[Previously published as
Change Your Diet and Change Your Life
Second paperback edition (revised and updated)
2012
ISBN: 978-1-907119-08-8]

Publisher: Tigmor Books
www.tigmorbooks.com

This book is dedicated to you the reader.
It is my sincere wish that the guidelines in this book help you
find the diet that truly works for you.

May you find health, happiness, and serenity.
You are unique—never doubt this.

Contents

Welcome

Are you fed up of being ill?

Have you, for as long as you can remember, been plagued by minor health problems such as headaches, skin rashes, cold and virus type symptoms, fleeting pains, bloating, sleeplessness, stomach upsets?

Have you never had a fully healthy skin?

Have you tried to lose weight and never succeeded or if you have lost weight have you put it on again?

Do you get recurring problems like joint and muscle pains, restless legs, fatigue, headaches, tics, rashes, depression, anxiety, tinnitus?

Have you had long periods of coping with everything and then suddenly become exhausted and has this happened more than once?

Do you feel tired after a full night's sleep?

Do you feel as if you have never totally been yourself?

Have you felt as if your life goes round in circles? You have periods of feeling okay when you get on with your life, make plans, see friends... Then you find the pace is speeding up, it seems that there's too much to do but you're still okay, coping.

Then suddenly, or so it appears, everything seems too much and you descend into feelings of despair and not coping—all you really want to do is withdraw. And, when it finally passes, do you feel confused and unsure of yourself?

Have you ever made a major change to your diet and, after an initial high, felt worse?

Do you frequently have stomach problems—wind, indigestion, constipation and/or diarrhoea?

Have you had bouts of anxiety, nervousness or depression for no apparent reason?

Does your vision fluctuate over the day—at times cloudy and then clear?

Do you have black shadows around your eyes or a feeling of grit beneath your eyelids?

Has a doctor, more than once, told you he can find nothing wrong or that there's nothing to worry about (the rash, pain, etc... will go away in time), or has he suggested your problem is stress related when you know it isn't?

If you have answered yes to more than one of the above questions then there is a strong likelihood that something you are eating is making you ill. You are in good company...

We change our diets, take supplements, exercise more and still we feel no better. So what is going wrong? It is my belief that the focus of most health care is fundamentally flawed. Rather than looking for the cause of our problems, doctors usually focus on treating the symptoms. We have come to accept this approach and to expect it, even demand it. We want the quick fix that will remove the pain, the rash or the depression but, sadly, without sorting out the cause the symptoms usually return.

If your diet is not the right one for you then you will not be as healthy as you could be both mentally and physically. By finding the diet that works for your body and mind you will change your life—you will experience fewer health problems, have more energy, an increased sense of well being and a return of hope and joy.

If this sounds far-fetched, I simply ask for your patience and time. Read on and you will discover for yourself the truth about how food can make you ill.

My story

Being constantly plagued by minor health problems had become a way of life for me. The crippling joint pain, the yo-yoing weight, the skin rashes, headaches, sinusitis, and tinnitus had become so usual that I had stopped seeing them as "illness" and accepted them as normal for me. What else could I do?

My diet was packed full of healthy fruit and vegetables. Visits to doctors invariably resulted in diagnoses of a virus, stress, wear and tear, or tiredness. There was, apparently, nothing wrong with me. I knew I wasn't as healthy as I could be but no matter what I did nothing changed. During this time I pretty much became an expert on relaxation techniques, meditation, healthy eating, stress management, alternative therapies and creative visualisation. Life, at times, did get easier but I was never fully well.

By the time I was in my late thirties, the problems had become serious. I was constantly ill and began experiencing episodes of severe debilitating tiredness and illness. According to the medical profession, there was nothing wrong with me that some fresh air, exercise and maybe a drop in weight wouldn't cure. But these measures did not work and my health got worse. I stopped being able to work and my life began to unravel.

Thankfully, I am a fighter and thankfully I had helped my husband "cure" his migraines and depression by identifying problems with grains, yeast, sugar and tyramine. Looking back I can only smile at how throughout that process it never once occurred to me that my own problems, mental as well as physical, could have their foundation in the food I was eating.

It was on a, sunny, day out in York that I finally made the connection. Sitting on the steps of the Minster exhausted after a very short walk and nursing a migraine, I watched people closely and came to the conclusion that the bloating I was experiencing and the translucent mottled skin I had developed were most definitely not normal. But what was wrong with me?

Biting into an apple my migraine raged even more ferociously and then receded leaving me with a severe low blood sugar problem. It was at that moment that I thought to myself that maybe, just maybe, some of my problems were being caused by food.

Within a few weeks of following an elimination diet I had made enormous progress. The weight began to disappear, the headaches stopped, my skin began to clear, my joints were mobile, my ears stopped ringing and my sinuses cleared. But what surprised me most of all were the changes in my behaviour and feelings.

The manic hyperactive energy followed by extreme fatigue, the mood swings, the inexplicable anxiety, tension, disorientation and confusion, the memory problems, and the extreme need to be alone all began to fade into the background. I had long ago decided that I had a personality defect probably caused by some event that was locked in my memory that I couldn't access. I was wrong, seriously wrong. These psychological and behavioural symptoms were all being caused by the food I was eating.

To cut a very long story short my health improved and I returned to work but a few months later began to re-experience problems. At this point it seemed that I was intolerant of nearly everything I ate and my diet was very restricted. I decided not give in but to carry out more research and eventually I discovered the information on food chemicals, salicylates in particular, which I needed. At last I had found the cause of my problems. The journey had been long, painful and extremely lonely but at last I had arrived at a reason and a "cure". I became far healthier than I had ever been.

My problems are not some medical oddity, quite the opposite. My research has shown me quite clearly that food intolerance can be the cause of many physical and mental health problems. It has also shown me that food as a cause is very rarely explored leaving many people to go throughout their lives suffering totally unnecessarily.

I believe that life is far too short to have its quality impaired by what we eat. I created the web site www.foodcanmakeyouill.co.uk and wrote this book to help others on their journey towards health. I do not believe that food intolerance is the cause of all problems but I do believe, and know, that for many a change in diet can truly change their lives.

The aims of this book

The aims of *The Food Intolerance Handbook* are:

- To provide you with an overview of the ways in which food can make people ill if they have a sensitivity to it.

- To explain the differences between food allergy and food intolerance.

- To outline a method, using the *Seven Step Plan*, that you can use to help you identify any food intolerance problems you may have.

- To introduce you to how food chemicals, natural and man-made, can cause problems.

- And, to introduce you to the concept of a truly healthy diet that works for you.

I wish you every success.
Sharla Race

Essential Information

The Food Intolerance Handbook has been written to provide information on the ways in which food can adversely affect the health of some individuals.

It is not my intention, nor should it be seen as being my intention, to provide medical advice or diagnosis. I am a researcher and writer, NOT a doctor.

As there are many possible causes of illness, it is essential that at all times you consult with your doctor or other medical practitioner. Any proposed changes to your diet should be discussed with your doctor or other medical practitioner before being started.

Under absolutely NO circumstances should you stop taking prescribed medication without the consent of your doctor.

It is my hope that you will find the information in this book useful and helpful but the responsibility for what you do with the information you read is completely your own.

Your health is the most precious resource you have—please look after yourself really well.

Sharla Race

1 You Are Unique

Yes, you are unique and in more ways than you can probably imagine. We live in an era that accepts differences in height, weight, body shape and personality without question yet assumes we all need the same type of food and the same amount of nutrients, to be healthy.

Biochemical individuality

In 1956, Dr Roger Williams, who discovered pantothenic acid (B5) and folic acid, coined the term "Biochemical Individuality". Biochemical individuality means that not only do we have a unique physical appearance but that internally we are also very different from each other.

Our internal organs are different sizes and the way they function varies. Some of us are deficient in certain enzymes such as those needed for digestion whilst others have these in abundance. Our ability to resist and fight disease varies. Some of us require vast amounts of certain nutrients whilst others don't, some feel pain more than others do and some of us are more likely to develop food intolerance and allergy problems than others.

Our genetic inheritance defines not only how we look but also how our bodies function internally at the level of every single cell. Before you start blaming your genes on everything, remember that other factors will also affect how healthy you are; these include your lifestyle, what you eat, the amount of exercise you take and your environment. But these only strengthen the argument for viewing each individual as exactly that—an individual.

So, although we are able to say that the body requires protein, minerals and vitamins we cannot say that you will function well on the same diet as me. Your needs will differ from mine and my needs will differ from yours. It is this fundamental uniqueness that provides the key to unravelling many baffling health problems.

The first step on the road to health is to embrace the idea that you are unique and that you may need to be treated differently than others with the same or similar symptoms. My focus in this book is to introduce you to the idea that eating the wrong diet could be impairing your physical and mental health.

The fact that you may have a problem with wheat, milk or a food chemical, such as salicylate, does not mean there is anything "wrong" with you. It is simply part of who you are— part of your own unique biochemical make-up. You may not find a cure but you will be able to find a solution by eliminating the food or reducing the amount that is consumed.

The myth of the healthy diet

It is a myth to suppose that there is such a thing as a single healthy diet that works for all. A healthy diet is a diet that works for you. You are unique and if you eat the wrong diet for you, even if it follows all the current healthy diet guidelines, you will not experience good health and you will probably have weight problems.

The current healthy diet guidelines generally suggest that you:

- Eat a variety of different foods.

- Eat the right amount to be a healthy weight.

- Eat plenty of foods rich in starch and fibre.

- Don't eat too many foods that contain a lot of fat.

- Don't have sugary foods and drinks too often.

- Don't eat too much salt.

- Look after the vitamins and minerals in your food.

- If you drink alcohol, drink within sensible limits.

The guidelines tend to focus around concepts of food pyramids, plates or tables which generally suggest that:

- Oils and fats should be used sparingly.

- Protein and dairy products should be eaten in moderation.

- At least five portions of fruit and vegetables should be eaten each day, with slightly more vegetables than fruit.

- Bread, cereal, rice, pasta and, sometimes, potatoes, should be the major part of the diet.

As a general guideline this may be adequate but it can never work for everyone. You could in fact follow these guidelines and be very unhealthy. For example, if you are intolerant of milk, gluten or wheat then you would not be able to eat the portions recommended in the dairy and grains sections without becoming seriously ill.

The detail within these guidelines changes virtually every year. I found it quite disconcerting that, at one point in the UK, the grains section included breakfast cereals, teacakes, crumpets and crackers all of which are potentially high in sugar, salt, refined grains and food additives. In the final analysis, these broad sets of guidelines can only ever be seen as that—broad guidelines. You will always need to adapt them to your own individual needs.

Do not see any dietary guidelines, unless they are avoiding an allergen that could kill you, as being cast in stone. Not only do the guidelines change virtually every year, the information we have on what is healthy and what isn't also changes. For example, evidence on dietary fat which has caused so much concern over the last few decades is contradictory. There have been times when all forms of fat were seen as potentially bad and whilst there is now more of a distinction between good and bad fats people remain confused and often interpret "low fat" as "no fat" which is potentially hazardous to their health.

Benton took a random sample of 7,076 British people and divided them into three groups depending on the amount of fatty foods that were eaten. The findings showed that reaction times of those eating higher amounts of fatty foods were quicker. The results did not differ across different age, sex or occupation groups.[1] Dr Ronald Krauss, chairman of the American Heart Association said that studies in healthy people show genetic differences in their response to low fat diets. It would seem that two thirds of the population would show only minimal benefit from a low fat diet and that for some it would be harmful.[2]

The focus on obtaining calories and nutrients from grains, meat and dairy products has also been called into question by the latest wave of interest in vegan diets and in raw foods. We all need protein, energy and nutrients from our food but how we obtain these will vary enormously. No single diet can be right for everyone.

Over the last forty years there has been an explosion of diets not just aimed at people wanting to lose weight but for general good health. They all come with the most amazing claims but if any of these worked for all of us wouldn't we all be healthier, and slimmer, than we currently are? By all means investigate the different diets on the market but don't be fooled into thinking that any one of them is 100% the right diet for you.

Success with some of these diets is often due to finding, by luck, one that excludes the foods that cause you a problem or provides you with the missing foods your body needs. For example, macrobiotic diets have worked wonderfully for some people but this could be because they have a sensitivity to the food chemical "solanine". All vegetables in the deadly nightshade family are excluded on a macrobiotic diet and all of these are high in solanine. Also, the diet relies on fresh food and has no preservatives and additives which further removes potentially troublesome elements from the diet.

The raw food diets work well for some because they increase the alkalinity in the body and make you feel great. For many they are a serious problem as most vegetables and fruit contain naturally occurring chemicals, such as salicylate, that some people are sensitive too. Stone Age diets remove grains, and often dairy products, from the diet as do many low carbohydrate diets. Could not the success of these be due to eliminating, two of the most common trouble makers, milk and wheat?

Weight loss diets that increase the fibre content of the diet may work because they are helping the individual to balance their blood sugar more and so prevent over eating. But for those with a grain sensitivity they do not work at all and in some cases lead to weight gain. Some people thrive on vegetarian diets whilst others become ill not because of the lack of meat protein but because they are consuming more dairy products than they can tolerate, have a sensitivity to lectins in beans, or are intolerant of certain grains or vegetables.

No "off the shelf" diet is going to work for everyone. Please do not think I am knocking these diets. I think the variety of them is a good thing and they are very useful for the people who can use them. But failing to improve, lose weight or being able to maintain one of these diets is not necessarily a sign that you have done something wrong, it is more likely that you have quite simply been trying to follow the wrong sort of diet for you.

It is strange that at this point in history we need guidelines on what to eat. Perhaps the greater choice and greater availability of food have clouded our own innate judgement as to what is healthy for us and what isn't but sadly guidelines can only ever be part of the story. You are going to have to take responsibility for your own diet.

If food was my problem surely I'd know, wouldn't I?

How I wish this could be true.

To doubt that there is a link between what you eat and your mental and physical health is a natural response. After all you eat food every day surely you would have noticed if you had a food related problem and surely, if it was a possibility, your doctor would have said something. If only it was that easy...

You could go throughout your whole life with your health being impaired without knowing that food was your problem or your doctor even suggesting it. The reason for this is the body's amazing ability to keep on going against the odds. Sadly, when the problem is not identified early on, the symptoms in the long term become more and more debilitating leading to depression, anxiety, fatigue and overall ill health. I shall try explaining what happens in a little more depth.

Your immune system is highly complex and amazing. It has many different layers of defence which are all designed to protect your body from harm whether it be from bacteria, viruses, parasites or toxins. It is a system that is spread throughout your body and it serves you well but it can get overworked. An exhausted immune system will not be able to protect you as well as it should.

One of the ways this exhaustion can come about is by a daily assault from food that is not right for you. Hans Selye in his book "The Stress of Life" describes how our bodies deal with prolonged bouts of stress. The description below is based loosely on his ideas.[3]

Stage One

At first, when it receives the food you have a problem with, your body will let you know that there is a problem—some symptoms will appear but these are often ignored, not noticed or happened when we were children so we don't remember them.

Stage Two

The body then goes into an acceptance phase. It adapts to the toxin and does its level best to keep you going. You may not experience very good health but you are managing.

Stage Three

Eventually it will reach the point of exhaustion. It can no longer deal with the onslaught and your health begins to break down. Mystery viruses, fatigue, minor problems, loss of zest etc... all begin to appear and you just never seem to feel well.

When stage three takes place will vary from individual to individual. For some it will take place in childhood, in others much later in life or as a result of illness or trauma. It is also not a one-off process. You may find that you become so ill that you have to rest for weeks or months and then you seem to be okay but actually you have returned to stage two and sooner or later will revisit stage three again.

The difficulty is that when stage three is reached you are often presenting a puzzling array of seemingly unrelated symptoms and it is not easy for any medical practitioner to recognise that food intolerance may be the root of the problem. This form of delayed hypersensitivity can involve a whole-body response involving several organ systems and leading to a chronic illness with recurring flu like symptoms. The array of resulting symptoms can be extremely puzzling. By my mid thirties I had such a long list of symptoms that I never presented them to a doctor for fear of being labelled a hypochondriac.

This breakdown in health does not take place overnight but can take a life-time to evolve. Usually in childhood there are symptoms of colic, eczema, nasal congestion, recurring ear infections and "growing" pains. The child seems fully well for only short periods of time. The pattern continues into adulthood with recurring bouts of a variety of symptoms such as nasal congestion, sore throats, generalised muscle aches and stiffness, abdominal pain and bloating, fatigue, weakness, an inability to think clearly and problems concentrating.

It is often the case that no specific physical cause can be found. People at some point acquire a label, either one of a number of syndromes such as chronic fatigue, fibromyalgia, irritable bowel, depression, panic disorder, or a single aspect is identified as the main problem such as migraine, rheumatic disease, asthma, Crohn's disease, urticaria, or arthritis. The presence of the hidden food problem is not identified and the individual continues to suffer.

Doctors, including Rowe and Randolph, have also identified a tension-fatigue syndrome, characterised by sensory and motor hyperactivity and/or sensory and motor fatigue, linked directly with food sensitivities. Once again, this condition does not appear overnight but at first occasionally bothers the individual then increases in occurrence and intensity leading the patient and doctor to a sense of desperation as nothing can be found to be wrong. The symptoms increase—tiredness after a full night's sleep, tiredness when not being particularly active, mental sluggishness, an inability to concentrate or get oneself going, possible depression, aching and sore muscles, bloating and so on. Studies by doctors who have accepted the existence of this syndrome have shown that the symptoms most generally go into remission when the offending foods are removed from the diet.

Food intolerance can occur at any age. It can be a short-term problem or a lifelong condition. If not identified early on it can lead to more serious problems in later life: for example, colitis in a child, which is caused by milk intolerance, can lead to Crohn's disease in adulthood.

It is also the case that any food can cause problems. Although some foods, like wheat and milk, have been identified as most likely to cause problems they are not the only culprits. **Any** food can cause your body and mind to be ill. You can be intolerant of any of the following:

♦ A complete food such as milk, soya, carrot, egg, pork, wheat, mushroom, chicken, apple.

♦ A naturally occurring chemical such as salicylate in many herbs, fruit and vegetables; tyramine in aged meat, cheeses and wine; purines in protein foods; amines in cooked foods; solanine in vegetables; or naturally occurring MSG (monosodium glutamate).

♦ An added ingredient that does not occur naturally in the food—such as a preservative, artificial sweetener, colouring, flavour or antioxidant.

♦ In a complex food, i.e. any processed food, you could be sensitive to any one of the ingredients. For example, in bread it is possible to react to wheat, preservatives, yeast, or flour improving agents.

Proven by many, not accepted by the majority

As you will discover, in the next chapter, there is an overwhelming amount of evidence that demonstrates how food can make you ill. So, why is the link between food and health, proven by many doctors, not accepted by the majority?

I put forward the following answers not as excuses but as a way of explaining the mechanism at work in traditional western medicine.

* Accepting food as a cause of illness is seen as too simplistic and would contradict accepted theories of disease causation put forward by highly respected members of the profession.

* There is always another promised wonder drug around the corner that, with media hype and marketing, overshadows research on links between food and illness.

* Increasing specialisation means doctors focus on a single set of symptoms rather than on the totality of the person.

* Treating symptoms rather than looking for causes is what doctors are taught to do.

* Doctors receive virtually no training in nutrition. The ones that come to accept the links between food and illness have often seen the effects of food intolerance on themselves, a relative or patient.

* The range of symptoms that can be caused by food intolerance is so vast that food intolerance would nearly always have to be considered and this is not seen as a valid use of a doctor's time—it is far easier, and saves time, to treat the symptom than to assist the individual in finding the cause.

- Assessing food intolerance is not something that can be done solely by the doctor—at some stage control must pass to the individual.

- There is still little understanding of how food intolerance and allergies can cause so many symptoms and this is unsettling to doctors used to relying on weighty tomes of scientific evidence.

- Little funding is available for research into the relationship between food and health. Drug research is more readily funded as pharmaceutical companies have a vested interest in the results. There is, quite simply, no profit to be made from understanding food intolerance.

- Research that requires the comparison of identical cases is virtually impossible in the area of food intolerance as what causes one individual to have, for example, migraines, will not necessarily cause migraines in another individual. Case studies are seen as being too individual specific and therefore are often ignored as evidence.

One of the other reasons is that doctors do not learn from their patients. Dr Mansfield, an advocate of the link between nutrition and arthritis, states that people who have had spectacular improvement in their arthritis have been met by disbelief when reporting their success with a change in diet to their GPs and rheumatologists. Their improvement in virtually all cases has been put down to "spontaneous remission". Dr Mansfield says: "These physicians, amazingly, seem uninterested by the patient's offer to re-eat the 'bad' foods and demonstrate an abrupt end to this 'spontaneous remission' for a few days."[4]

Other doctors, including Philpott, Mackarness, Mumby, Randolph, and Rowe, have been equally amazed at how findings on links between nutrition and health have, rather than being embraced, been ignored. Professor Jonathon Brostoff, Professor of Allergy and Environmental Health, University College, London, said that re-education of doctors was essential. "The education system does not even mention nutrition, let alone food intolerance. We do not have a body of doctors who have learned about the role of food and diet in health."[5]

During the course of the research for this book, I have come to appreciate the difficulty faced by doctors and researchers in scientifically establishing the role of food in illness. Thankfully, with appropriate tests, allergies can now be more easily recognised but food intolerance continues to cause problems. This will become easier when the various mechanisms by which food affects individuals become known and defined. Research in the area of food additives and the problems caused by naturally occurring food chemicals is taking place but is fraught with difficulties for the following reasons.

- Little is still known about why some individuals have problems with eliminating these substances from their bodies.

- Most of these substances are cumulative in the body and this can make testing extremely difficult.

- The symptoms produced vary in type and intensity from individual to individual.

- ◆ Tolerance levels are individual specific.

- ◆ Challenging with a single dose often produces a negative result.

This inability to explain why food "x" causes symptom "y" and the fact that any food can cause any symptom leaves many doctors sceptical and resistant to exploring food intolerance as the cause of illness. Scepticism is healthy but total dismal is ignorance and the result is that millions of people are denied the help that they need. Suffering continues and the cost of health care keeps on rising.

It was interesting reviewing the research more than ten years after this book was first published as nothing had changed:

- ◆ Scepticism about the role of food intolerance in causing health problems remains quite common

- ◆ Medical journals still contain case studies presented by doctors who are astounded that for at least one of their patients food was actually the cause of their illness.

- ◆ Research papers are still being written that describe how some individuals make amazing recoveries when their diets are changed and that perhaps other doctors should consider testing for food sensitivities.

What has changed is the way each of us, as individuals, can access information. The internet has enabled us to explore and find out more about a diagnosis we have been given and to discuss with others ways forward that might help us.

One cannot fault the drive for medical advances to prevent or cure diseases that cause so many deaths such as cancer and heart disease but ignoring the host of more minor complaints that people continuously suffer from is criminally insane. It is time health organisations and professionals recognised that avoiding certain foods and additives can greatly improve, even cure, a person's condition, improve their quality of life and help prevent more serious illness.

As Gaby in his paper on the role of hidden food allergy and food intolerance in chronic diseases says: "Food allergy is an important and frequently overlooked cause of (or triggering factor for) a wide range of chronic, physical and mental disorders. Routine use of elimination diets in clinical practice can greatly increase the response rate in many difficult-to-treat medical conditions."[6]

Doctors' indifference to the role of nutrition in illness is perhaps nowhere best seen than in the disregard for evidence that shows that hospitalised people are frequently provided with nutritionally deficient diets. A few examples follow:

- Todd et al found that the daily energy, protein, iron and vitamin intake of people on different wards of an English hospital were less than those recommended for healthy adults.[7]

- Allison found that treatable malnutrition could be occurring in up to 25% of hospital patients and that nutritional status may also deteriorate during a prolonged stay. Suggestions were made that hospital managers had a positive policy towards nutritional care, that catering services recognised and addressed the problem and that, for optimal success, a skilled nutrition team was necessary and cost effective.[8]

- Nevett found that malnutrition is a common problem amongst hospitalised people and that this leads to an increased risk of mortality and morbidity.[9]

- The development of malnutrition whilst in hospital is the result of changes in diet, nutrition not being seen as a high priority, common hospital practices, and lack of knowledge of people's previous nutritional state is the conclusion reached by Edwards in a comprehensive overview of malnutrition in hospital people.[10]

I find these type of studies distressing. Surely, during a stay in hospital, you should be able to expect the best possible care and that this should include an adequate and nutritious diet.

In 1999, a study by the Nuffield Trust in the UK, found that 40% of adults in hospital were undernourished and many others become so during their time in hospital. The report recommended that food provision be considered as part of clinical care rather than a "hotel" function.[11] The situation did not improve and in 2008 a report warned that malnutrition was still common in NHS hospitals and that the problem had increased by 85% over the past 10 years. By the way, this problem isn't restricted to the UK—surveys elsewhere consistently find that about 20% of patients in general hospitals are malnourished.[12]

The role of food in health is being overlooked by those very people responsible for our health and who produce the guidelines for healthy eating. Just what message are they sending out if their healthy eating guidelines are not implemented in hospitals?

By ignoring nutrition and the role that food intolerance plays in illness, doctors are closing the door on health for a great many people. If someone presents at a doctor's surgery with a recurring rash and headaches that individual's body is undergoing stress and if it is not dealt with adequately their immune system will suffer. If an ointment and pain relief are prescribed then the symptoms may abate but the problem will still remain—prescribing a different ointment and higher strength pills will still not solve the problem.

The more stress and damage we do to our finely tuned immune systems the harder it will be for them to deal with an invasive disease or illness. Modern medicine has become focused on signs and symptoms, and drugs and treatments to "cure" them. The approach by doctors has become standardised and narrow, overlooking (usually not even considering) the unique aspects of an individual's condition.

Finding appropriate help has become expensive and exhausting and it is a tragedy that many people are unable to get the help they need. The food we eat, and the environment we live in, can never be ignored. For many people, an exploration of these would lead to an end to unnecessary suffering. And food intolerance does cause suffering—not just rashes and headaches but, if not identified, a lifetime of chronic ill health can ensue.

If doctors can't help us we need to educate ourselves and force them to "hear" us. I know you may have great difficulty finding appropriate help but at least through this book, and others, you will have more information to guide you and help you guide your helpers. We need to take more responsibility for our own health.

Why you need to involve your doctor

You may be asking yourself why I insist on you involving your doctor when so many have little experience of this field. Quite simply—illness is complex and has many causes and I do not want you to undergo any additional unnecessary suffering. If all other causes of your problem have been eliminated and your doctor does not want you to try dietary changes you can always change doctors.

As awareness increases more help will become available and there are, currently, doctors who are experts in this field and others who have a more open mind than some of their colleagues. It is important to obtain the appropriate help as testing for allergies is always safest when carried out by trained medical staff—anaphylactic reactions can lead to death.

I must stress that involving your doctor is even more important if you are suffering from any mental health problems, whether diagnosed or not, as the reactions that can take place when testing foods can be extreme. In these instances, testing of foods must be done with medical supervision.

References

[1] Benton D. Lipids and cognitive functioning. In: Hillbrand M and Spitz R T (eds). Lipids and Human Behaviour. American Psychological Assoc 1996.

[2] BMJ News. Very low fat diets may harm some people. BMJ 1998;316:517.

[3] Selye H. The Stress of Life. McGraw-Hill rev ed, 1984.

[4] Mansfield J. Arthritis, Allergy, Nutrition and the Environment. Thorsons 1995.

[5] Brostoff J. BBC News on-line Tuesday October 13 1998. http:\\www.bbc.co.uk.

[6] Gaby AR. The role of hidden food allergy/intolerance in chronic disease. Altern Med Rev 1998;3(2):90-100.

[7] Todd E A et al. What do patients eat in hospital. Human Nutr Ampi Nutr 1984;38A:294-97.

[8] Allison SP. The management of malnutrition in hospital. Proc Nutr Soc 1996;55(3):855-62.

[9] Nevett G. Malnutrition of the hospitalised patient-assessment of provision of diet and dietary intake. EDTNA ERCA J 1997;23(4):22-4.

[10] Edwards SL. Malnutrition in hospital patients: where does it come from? Br J Nurs 1998;7(16):954-8,971-4.

[11] Davis AM, Bristow A. Managing Nutrition in Hospital. Nuffield Trust Report, 1999.

[12] Lean M, Wiseman M. Malnutrition in hospitals. BMJ. 2008 Feb 9;336(7639):290.

2 Food Can Make You Ill

It is a common misconception that adverse reactions always occur within minutes of eating the problem food. The following list shows the full range of ways in which food intolerance can manifest itself:

- An immediate reaction such as a rash, breathing problems, generalised swelling, mouth ulcers.

- A delayed reaction, causing physical symptoms or behavioural changes that can occur anywhere from a few hours to a few days after eating the food.

- No immediate reaction but episodic bouts of recurring illness—usually focused on one area whether it be the joints, nose, skin or digestive system.

- Recurring bouts of general malaise and flu-like or non-specific symptoms.

- A general sense of never really feeling well with no noticeable starting point.

- A history of recurring illness—specific and non-specific often leading to periods of crisis in health, frequently starting in childhood and continuing into adulthood.

- A sudden down turn in health after serious illness, drug treatment, major stress or trauma.

The result of presenting these symptoms to a doctor is often treatment for a viral infection, depression or stress. As the condition progresses a label may be given—irritable bowel syndrome, arthritis, chronic fatigue syndrome etc... At this point the search for answers usually stops and the search for solutions begins. But if the diagnosis is wrong then the solution will never wholly appear.

There may be improvement but the problem never goes away and the patient becomes the label and may, as time progresses, move on to acquiring even more labels. If you have been diagnosed as having a condition your first step on the road to recovery could very well be to throw out the label you have been given.

Still in doubt? In 1976 Dr Richard Mackarness, writing of the UK, estimated that "30 per cent of people attending GPs have symptoms traceable exclusively to food and chemical allergy; 30 per cent have symptoms partly traceable to this cause, and the remaining 40 per cent have symptoms that are unrelated to allergy."[1]

Dr Coca, in 1945, estimated that as many as 90% of Americans had one or more food allergies.[2] In the 1970s Dr Mandell estimated that fifty to eighty per cent of the daily medical practice of most doctors was the "result of allergy and chemical susceptibility".[3] It is highly unlikely that this has changed.

Symptoms

Some general indicators of food being a problem include:

- Feeling unwell all over.

- Fluctuating weight.

✓ ◆ Occasional swelling of face, hands, feet and more generally.

✓ ◆ Persistent stomach problems.

✓ ◆ Persistent tiredness not helped by sleep or rest.

✓ ◆ Sudden changes from feeling well to unwell.

✓ ◆ Sudden tiredness or chills after eating.

To give you an idea of the type of problems that food intolerance can cause, lists of symptoms are given below. Each of the symptoms and conditions has been found, in some individuals, to be caused by food. Please do not assume that just because your symptom or condition is listed that food is the cause—check it out with your doctor first. The purpose of these lists is solely to give you an idea of the overwhelming range of symptoms and illness that can be caused by eating food that is not right for you.

Many things can affect the severity and intensity of symptoms. For some people the amount of the food or food chemical may be a significant factor. For others it can be overall health, the amount of sleep they've had or the level of different hormones in their system. Hormonal changes, in both men and women, can affect reactions.[4]

Physical problems

A wide range of physical problems have been associated with food intolerance and they include:

Abdominal pain, aching muscles and joints, acne, addictions, arthritis, asthma, athlete's foot.

Bad breath, bedwetting, blackouts, bloating, blood sugar problems, blurred vision, breast pain.

Catarrh, Chronic Fatigue Syndrome, coated tongue, colitis, constant hunger, constipation, crawling sensation on skin.

Diarrhoea, difficulty in swallowing, dizziness.

Eczema, excessive thirst, excessive or no sweating.

Fatigue, feeling drained, flushes, food cravings,

Frequent need to urinate, frequent sore throat.

Gall bladder problems, gritty feeling in eyes.

Headaches, heavy body odour, high/low blood pressure, hives.

Indigestion (recurring), insomnia, Irritable Bowel Syndrome, itching, itchy and red ears.

Joint pain, stiffness and swelling.

Lethargy.

Menstrual problems, metallic taste, migraine, mouth ulcers, muscle aches, cramps, spasm and tremor, muscle weakness.

Nausea.

Palpitations, persistent cough, poor balance, post-nasal drip, pre-menstrual problems.

Racing pulse, rashes, recurring ear infections, restless legs syndrome.

Sensitivity to light and/or noise, sinusitis, sleep disturbances, sore tongue, stiff neck, styes, sore burning eyes.

Temperature fluctuations, thrush, tics, tinnitus.

Urticaria.

Vertigo.

Watering eyes, weight problems, wheezing.

Whilst this is a frighteningly long list of the ways in which food can make you ill, I personally find it even more worrying that food can also seriously affect your mental health.

Mind, emotions and behaviour

The mind, emotions, and behaviour can all be affected adversely simply by what you eat. The types of problems have included:

Accident proneness, anger for no apparent reason, anxiety, attention deficit hyperactivity disorder.

Behavioural problems, blankness, brain fogging.

Changes in handwriting, clumsiness, confusion.

Delusions, depression, detached or unreal feeling, difficulty waking up, disorientation, dyslexia.

Feelings of disassociation, feeling tense and ill at ease, fidgeting.

Hallucinations, hearing without comprehension, hyperactivity.

Inability to think clearly, indifference, irritability.

Learning difficulties.

Math and spelling errors, memory loss, mental exhaustion, mood swings.

Panic attacks, phobias, poor concentration, poor self-image, poor memory.

Reading problems, restlessness.

Slow processing information, slurred speech, stammering, suicidal feelings.

Uncontrollable rage.

Weepiness, withdrawn.

Many people are surprised to discover that behaviour, emotions and feelings can be determined by the food we eat but the cells in the brain are just as at risk as any other in the body. Consider how alcohol affects you and how it affects others differently. The same principle applies to food.

The bloodstream carries molecules of chemicals, natural and artificial, throughout the body. In the brain, these chemicals interfere with the chemical and electrical functioning of the brain cells and so affect our thoughts, feelings and behaviour. It can take a very small amount of a chemical, that your body sees as toxic, to produce an unwanted effect. Some additives and natural food chemicals, such as salicylate, are very similar in structure to some of the brain's neurotransmitters and, when these are wrongly identified by the body, internal chaos begins. Emotional factors are, most definitely, not the only explanation for mental disturbances.

Rinkel, Randolph and Zeller showed that removing foods, and then reintroducing them into the diet, could lead to the disappearance and subsequent reappearance of a variety of "psychological" symptoms including catatonia, delusions, depression, feeling drugged, hallucinations, headaches and paranoia.[5]

Dr Mumby writes that he has seen allergy (food and environmental) lead to "heightened sexual feelings, murderous assault, schizophrenic psychosis, woolly thinking, hallucination, hyperactivity, depression, anxiety, learning difficulties, dyslexia and autism."[6]

Speer in his book *Allergy of the Nervous System*, published in 1970, presents evidence that shows that emotional and neurological symptoms arising from allergies have been recorded since the 1920s.[7] In fact, in 1905, Francis Hare, an Australian doctor, wrote *Food Factor in Disease* in which he gave numerous examples of people whose symptoms include "mental problems" that were caused by various foods.[8]

Dr Randolph, at the time of writing his book, had treated about 20,000 people for food allergies and related problems having dealt with "every kind of chronic illness on an allergic basis". About 37.5 per cent of these people were primarily suffering from "mental problems"; many were helped significantly often when conventional treatments had failed. He says that allergy can be responsible for a "host of so-called mental problems, including some cases of what looks like outright psychoses".[9]

Dr Philpott, in his book on Brain Allergies, provides us with numerous examples including:

- hyperactivity in a child being caused by string beans;

- violent anger in a woman that was triggered by oranges;

- sensitivity to wheat in a seventeen year old who had been classed as mentally ill for three years;

- watermelons leading to depression and irritability in a twelve year old;

- manic depression being caused by milk in a thirty year old patient.

Dr Philpott cites many other cases where people's "psychological" problems have in fact turned out to be reactions to food, chemicals in the environment, preservatives and additives, non-caking agents in table salt, and chlorinated water.[10]

What surprises, and saddens, me greatly is that this information is not more widely available and that it is not embraced by the medical profession. You are still more likely to be given pills, hospitalised or told there is nothing wrong with you than have your diet and environment examined for clues to your condition.

There is now an acceptance and understanding that certain drugs will have side effects that produce a change in behaviour. In fact some drugs are designed to do exactly that—change how you behave and feel. If we accept that drugs do this, often with little understanding of how, why can we not accept that food and the chemicals within food can do the same?

Let's just briefly look at two hypothetical examples. I am taking more time to explore the links between food and the mind because this is a seriously neglected area of study and you need to know that it is not only your body that is at risk from poisoning by the food you eat.

In our first example, twenty-six year old Josh complains of being tired all the time. He is irritable, has no energy and little interest in anything. He is a busy individual with many responsibilities and says he is feeling under stress yet has previously coped quite adequately with far busier and more demanding times in his life. He also has fleeting joint pains, migraines and a recurring rash. A battery of tests identify no physical problem and the doctor is likely to agree with the diagnosis of "stress". Josh may also be prescribed exercise to help joint mobility, pain killers for the migraine, and ointment for the rash. None of which will help identify and then treat the cause of the problem.

In our second example, forty-five year old Carol has developed agoraphobia. Her husband died a year ago and she now finds herself unable to leave the house. Prior to his death and for the first two months after his death she had no symptoms of agoraphobia. The most obvious diagnosis would be that the agoraphobia was brought on by the bereavement and to recommend a course of counselling. But would something different emerge if Carol was asked about any other changes in her life?

In both the above cases it is easy to see how the diagnoses were arrived at but what if Josh had quite simply reached a time in his life when his body just could no longer cope with the diet he was eating—maybe his sensitivity to wheat, which he eats at every meal, had reached crisis point.

What if Carol's problem was that her husband had been the cook and her diet had changed dramatically from homemade meals to take-outs and microwave dinners. The end result being that she was taking in additives and MSG to such an extent that they were affecting her brain, increasing her anxiety and preventing her from leaving the house? There have been studies (some are mentioned in Martin's book *The Sickening Mind*[11]) that show the immune function of the bereaved partner is diminished in the weeks after the death. This reduction in function could have been the key factor in stopping her body processing the cocktail of chemicals she was now eating. She could in fact always have been sensitive to MSG or an additive. Had she ever in the past experienced a similar problem?

Five, ten or fifteen minute consultations will never provide these answers. If you truly want to get well, you need to be an active participant in the process. Your doctor only knows your symptoms not you. Food intolerance can cause problems across the behavioural spectrum from manic "happy" behaviour to severe depression.

We seemed to have reached a point in our history where we too easily blame our mental states on inherent personality flaws or stress. Yet it could just be what you are eating. I had certainly never experienced the calm that I now have until I changed my diet. I thought that my anxiety, mood swings and hyperactivity were just part of who I was. They were not—they were only symptoms arising from substances that my body saw as toxins.

Perhaps the most dangerous diagnosis of the modern age, aside from "stress" is that of psychosomatic illness. This is when no physical cause can be found for the symptoms you have and the doctor therefore assumes that they must be being induced by your mental state. This assumption becomes a diagnosis that may lead to some form of talking therapy, a suggestion to reduce stress or no action at all. All three of these will be totally ineffective in relieving symptoms in the long term. If your body is being poisoned by the food you eat, or the chemicals in your environment, then you will continue to be ill until these are removed and you begin to recover.

Dr Philpott writes: "According to Randolph—and my experience bears this out—more than half of the so-called psychosomatic reactions are in reality undiagnosed allergic reactions."[12] And Rapaport suggests that: "If mental illness caused by allergies were recognised more, and emotional factors not always sought to explain mental disturbances, a great deal of time and money could be saved, and people's mental conditions eliminated."[13]

Just living...

Food intolerance does not just lead to physical and mental symptoms. It affects all areas of your life including your appearance, relationships, work, leisure activities, and self-esteem. The ways in which it can affect your appearance include:

- You can look fatter and flabbier than the "real" you actually is. Bloating/swelling can occur on your face, legs, ankles and feet, around your abdomen, thighs and buttocks.

- You could spend a fortune on products trying to clear your cellulite with no success when all you need to is change your diet.

- Your skin will probably not be at its best. It could be too oily, dry, or covered in a rash or spots that you just cannot clear.

- Your eyes could have a discharge, be bloodshot or cloudy, seem very small due to swollen eyelids, feel grainy and tired. At times, your vision may be blurred and your eyes could be light sensitive.

- Your lips could be cracked, sore and swollen. Your tongue may be coated, sore and swollen and your mouth plagued with ulcers. And, regardless of how thorough a dental hygiene programme you have, you could have bad breath.

- Your nose could be swollen, constantly running, itchy or red in colour.

- Your hair, no matter what you do with it, could be lank, excessively dry or oily.

- If you are constantly feeling ill you probably look tired, miserable and, maybe, even sad or anxious.

- Clothes and shoes won't always fit—one day they'll be fine, the next too tight and uncomfortable.

Some of the other ways in which food intolerance can have an impact on your life include:

- ◆ Limiting the activities you can do due to, for example, fatigue and joint pain.

- ◆ Work can become increasingly stressful when you are plagued with problems due to brain fogging that affect your ability to concentrate and lead to memory problems.

- ◆ You may have been passed over at work because of excessive time away due to sickness. You may even have had to give up your career.

- ◆ Relationships can be put under serious strain by constantly having to deal with a partner's seemingly unexplainable bouts of low energy, forgetfulness, irritability, depression, mood swings, seeming distant and far away, anxiety, and obsessive behaviour.

Not all illness is food related but ...

As the studies below demonstrate, it can be the sole cause or a major factor for many individuals and in a wide range of conditions.

Without food we would die and given this crucial role that food plays in our lives it does seem strange that its role in illness (and health) is not more fully acknowledged and used in treatments.

The cost to the individual is enormous—loss of health and a deterioration in the quality of life. The financial cost to society of continuously treating recurring conditions is enormous yet treatments relying on food avoidance cost virtually nothing, except time, in comparison. This is highlighted in an experiment with phlebitis sufferers.

> Rea et al divided twenty individuals with recurrent intractable non-traumatic phlebitis into two groups, matching them for age and severity. The control group continued on their usual anticoagulant treatment, bed rest and support hose. The other group were placed in an "Environmental Control Unit" where all the air, water and food could be controlled. All medication, for this group, was stopped. In eight out of ten, of this group, the phlebitis was found to be triggered by food sensitivities and inhaled chemicals such as formaldehyde.

> In a five year follow up study this group showed two 48 hour episodes of phlebitis cleared by home bed rest and food abstinence. In contrast, the control group had more than sixty episodes of phlebitis at home and forty one episodes in hospital. Medical costs in these comparable groups showed a differential of $20 per person in the Environmental Control Unit treatment versus more than $20,000 per person in the control group over the five year follow up.[14]

The cost to society is not just financial, it is also a massive loss of work time, creativity and energy. Changing your diet can change *your* life and, by doing so, affects everyone you come into contact with and everything that you do.

In October 2000, the British government apologised for the mistakes and delays that took place during the BSE crisis. Wrong advice was given to the public about the dangers of eating beef and people died, and continue to do so, from the human variant CJD. It took 15 years for this apology to materialise and the report cast serious doubts on our ability to believe government reassurances and advice on food safety. What struck me at the time of this report was that it had taken deaths and very specific scientific proof that these were linked with mad cow disease before any real action was taken.

The long term debilitating effects of food substances such as additives and artificial sweeteners are not visible in the same way but this does not mean they do not exist. Will sufferers ever receive an apology? Will we ever be totally able to rely on government advice? Can we truly trust others with our health?

If you think that food, in some form, might be affecting your health please do not let yourself be dismissed by health care professionals. Persist—it is your life, your health. You might be wrong but you might be right. There comes a time when you have to set the advice aside, find out more for yourself and listen to your body. There is only one person who is going to take your health totally seriously and that is you.

Evidence

More than 2000 years ago Hippocrates said "Let your food be your medicine and your medicine be your food". He, like many doctors down the centuries, accepted the link between food and illness. In the twelfth century, Maimonides stated that no illness that could be treated by diet should be treated in any other way. They understood that simple changes to the diet were sometimes all that was needed.

Despite overwhelming amounts of evidence accumulated by modern day doctors and researchers, this is not a view that has been embraced by Western medicine. The search remains focused on finding "cures" that have nothing to do with diet and doctors prescribe treatments that relieve symptoms rather than cure them. Yet, it seems that the basic truth that food can make you ill and a change in diet can make you well is continuously being rediscovered by doctors.

It is a sad fact that many people discover that they are food intolerant without the help of a doctor and when they present this information to the doctor they are not believed. As much as I find this highly annoying, I also find it understandable. Vickers and Zollman found that, although nutrition as a science has always been part of conventional medicine, doctors are not taught, and therefore do not practise, much in the way of nutritional therapeutics.[15]

Dieticians in conventional settings tend to work mainly with particular patient groups such as those with diabetes, obesity, digestive, or cardiovascular risk factors. Apart from the treatment of severe nutritional deficiencies and rare metabolic disorders, other nutritional interventions generally fall outside the mainstream and have therefore come to be seen as complementary medicine.

Also, if you have never witnessed for yourself a food reaction then you will be sceptical. Doctors who begin to use elimination diets, a method of testing for food intolerance, are also at first taken aback at the range of symptoms and the number of foods that their patients claim they have a reaction too. But, in the words of Dr Mansfield: "People do not want to react adversely particularly to their favourite foods, and are more likely to ignore a minor reaction to a favourite food than to invent reactions that do not exist."[16] Obvious really.

In 1998 the British Allergy Research Foundation stated that there is now abundant evidence that conditions such as irritable bowel syndrome and asthma are linked to food allergies but that the connection is still not recognised by many GPs with the result that many people suffer years of misery before they are properly diagnosed (if they ever are). They estimated that one in four people suffers from some form of allergic disease and found evidence that food intolerance causes or exacerbates conditions such as asthma, migraine, nasal congestion, eczema, hyperactivity, irritable bowel syndrome and Crohn's disease. In respect of Crohn's disease, 50% feel better when a particular food is eliminated from their diet. By 2012, they were estimating that one in three Britons had an allergy.[17]

Studies looking at statistics in 2006 found that, since 1990, admissions to hospital, in the UK, for anaphylaxis have increased by 700%, for food allergy by 500%, for urticaria by 100%, and for angioedema by 40%.[18] In 1999 the BBC ran a mini series called "Allergy Alert". Their review of studies in different western populations showed at least 15% of the population to be allergic which in Britain means around eight million people.[19]

French Allergy researchers reported that multiple food intolerance in infants and young children is increasing. Moneret-Vautrin et al estimate that more than 40% of infants less than one year old could be affected. The most common food allergens are milk, egg, soya and wheat but other foods are also implicated.[20] In the US, the Centre for Disease Control estimated that in 2007, approximately 3 million children under the age of eighteen were reported to have a food or digestive allergy in the previous year. They also noted that from 1997 to 2007, the prevalence of reported food allergy increased 18% among children under the age of eighteen.[21]

Figures vary according to the food and country, and the collection of statistics on allergies is not carried out in the same way in all countries. I could continue quoting figures but at best they are estimates and do not give a true picture of the ways in which food affects health. Part of the problem is with definitions. The focus of these statistics is usually allergies that can be observed objectively using scientific methods of testing. Yet, food intolerance which causes problems for countless people cannot be measured in this way.

Some doctors when quoting statistics will estimate far greater numbers because they are aware of food intolerance but others don't. So what is the truth? At the moment we don't know. I suspect that the number of people with food intolerance problems is far greater than ever suspected but until methods of identifying and classifying these cases is carried out we will not know for definite.

Before continuing, I would like to extend a very big thank you to the doctors, scientists, researchers and the individuals who have participated in the studies outlined below. Without this type of research there would be no hope at all of the medical profession exploring the role of food in illness and health. Maybe, just maybe, we are at stage three in the development of a new medical idea as put forward as a "joke" in Dr Mumby's book *The Complete Guide to Food Allergies and Environmental Illness:*[22]

1. You are mad.
2. There might be something in it.
3. There might be something in it but where is the proof?
4. Of course, we knew all along.

The purpose of this section is to highlight some of the research that has been carried out that has identified food as the cause of ill health. It is by no means comprehensive, there are thousands of articles out there, but is presented here to give you an idea of the work being done and also to show you that many doctors do recognise that food can make you ill.

These are very brief summaries of just a small proportion of the studies and reports that can be found in the medical literature on the links between food and specific health conditions.

Acute Pancreatitis

Matteo and Sarles report on two cases of acute recurrent pancreatitis, lasting for eight and ten years, characterised by acute abdominal pain. They concluded that both cases were due to food allergy and that food allergy could, for some people, be the cause of acute recurrent pancreatitis. The problem foods, for these people, were beef, milk, potato, fish, and eggs.[23]

A twenty-three year old with recurring episodes of acute pancreatitis and other symptoms (including red patches on the face, generalised itching and diarrhoea) found that root of the problem was cow's milk.[24] Another case of acute pancreatitis was found to be caused by an allergy to kiwi fruit.[25]

Anorexia Nervosa

Stolze et al present the case of a woman who had suffered from weight loss, stomach problems, headaches, flushing and bronchial asthma for several years. The diagnosis had been anorexia nervosa.

After following a diet low in histamine the woman experienced weight gain and an improvement in all her other symptoms. It therefore appears that the condition she had in fact been suffering from was histamine intolerance.[26]

Arthritis

Links between food and arthritis have been recorded in the medical literature as far back as 1917. Dr John Mansfield, a

British doctor specialising in allergy and nutrition, states that most "forms of arthritis are environmentally and nutritionally induced."[27]

Hicklin et al administered an elimination diet to twenty two people with rheumatoid arthritis. Twenty of the individuals (91%) noticed an improvement in their symptoms, and nineteen found that certain foods repeatedly caused a return or aggravation of symptoms.[28]

Ratner et al studied fifteen women and eight men with rheumatoid or psoriatic arthritis. The people were instructed to remove dairy products and beef from their diet. Seven people improved. The authors concluded that a diet free of dairy products and beef was of value in lactase-deficient women with seronegative rheumatoid arthritis or psoriatic arthritis.[29]

Panush et al outlined a detailed case study of a fifty-two year old woman whose inflammatory arthritis was severely exacerbated by milk.[30]

Beri et al prescribed an "elimination and rechallenge" diet to twenty seven people with rheumatoid arthritis. Of the fourteen who completed the diet program, ten (71%) showed significant clinical improvement.[31]

Darlington treated seventy people with rheumatoid arthritis by identifying and eliminating symptom-provoking foods. Of these seventy, 19% remained well and did not require any medications during follow-up periods (ranging from 1.5 to 5 years). The foods that most commonly caused symptoms were: corn (56%), wheat (54%), bacon/pork (39%), oranges (39%), milk, oats (37% each), rye (34%), egg, beef, coffee (32% each), malt (27%), cheese, grapefruit (24% each), tomato (22%), peanuts, cane sugar (20% each), and butter, lamb, lemon, and soy (17% each).[32]

Many studies deal with rheumatoid arthritis but there is also a large amount of anecdotal evidence that links gouty arthritis with a diet too high in purines, and arthritic and joint pain, more generally, has been linked with a diet too high in solanine.

See also *Joint Pain.*

Asthma

Asthma is a condition that has been studied extensively and individual foods, food additives and food chemicals have all been found to be responsible for some individuals' asthma.

Businco et al state that, currently, wheezing is considered unusual in food intolerant people but that cases of food-induced asthma have been observed particularly in children.[33] Food allergy may trigger allergic respiratory symptoms through two main routes: ingestion or inhalation.

Some examples of the available research linking food sensitivity with asthma are given below.

- Stevenson and Simon,[34] Stenius and Lemola,[35] and Freedman[36] all found that sensitivity to food additives such as metabisulfites, tartrazine, sodium benzoate, and sulphur dioxide acted as trigger factors for asthma in some individuals.

- Pelikan and Pelikan-Filipek found that out of one hundred and seven people with perennial asthma, sixty (56%) had an asthmatic response to ingestion of one or more foods.[37]

- Allen et al found that MSG could provoke asthma and noted that the reaction to MSG was dose dependent and may be delayed up to twelve hours, after ingestion, making recognition difficult.[38]

- Eriksson found that 24% of adults with bronchial asthma and/or allergic hay fever

- had some kind of food sensitivity—hazelnut, apple and shellfish being the most common.[39]

- Rousquet et al identified that between 7 and 29% of asthma sufferers had a milk sensitivity.[40]

- Genton et al challenge tested individuals with asthma with a number of compounds including acetylsalicylic acid, sodium benzoate, sulfur dioxide, sodium glutamate and tartrazine. Over half of those in the study were found to be intolerant of at least one compound. For some of the group, a diet free of additives resulted in a marked improvement within five days.[41]

- Pirson et al reported that a person working in a factory producing inulin from chicory developed rhinoconjuctivitis and asthma to the dust of dry chicory roots and oral allergy syndrome to raw fruits and vegetables. A provocation test with dry chicory induced acute rhinoconjuctivitis and an immediate asthmatic response. [42]

Attention Deficit Hyperactivity Disorder

Kidd explains that the exact aetiology of ADHD, which often persists into adulthood, is unknown but that adverse responses to food additives and food sensitivities do play a role in the condition for some individuals.[43] The pioneer in this field was Dr Feingold who in the 1970s identified sensitivity to food additives, and often salicylates, as the cause of hyperactivity in up to 50% of children so diagnosed.[44]

Although Feingold has been much criticised, it is the case that links between food and behaviour had been previously noted. As early as 1922, Shannon had published information on the successful treatment of children with hyperactivity and learning disorders using an elimination diet; 30-50% of children improved.[45]

More recently, Schardt reviewed more than twenty double-blind studies that examined whether food dyes or ordinary foods worsened behaviour in children with ADHD or other behavioural problems. In the majority of the studies, the behaviour of some children worsened after consumption of food dyes or improved on an additive-free diet. Individual foods also caused problems for some children.[46]

Kidd tells us that Feingold's original case histories covered 1,200 cases in which food additives were linked to behavioural and learning disorders, and implicated a vast number of additives yet subsequent research attempting to verify his work has focused on less than a dozen additives. "It is interesting to note that studies conducted in non-US countries produced results markedly more favourable to the Feingold interpretation, and that most of the US investigations were sponsored by a corporate food lobby group, the Nutrition Foundation." [47]

As Boris[48] demonstrates, studies that eliminate a single additive tend to show little improvement whilst those eliminating a wider range are a great deal more successful.[49,50] Up to 88% of ADHD children react to these substances in sublingual challenge testing, but in blinded studies no child reacted to these alone.[51]

Carter et al found that on an elimination diet, fifty nine out of seventy eight children with hyperactive behaviour problems improved.[52] Data from two double-blind studies indicated that 73-76% of ADHD children respond favourably to food elimination diets.[53] Maintenance on even more-restricted, low-antigen (oligoantigenic) diets raised the success rate as high as 82%. Invariably in these studies, reintroduction of the offending foods led to reappearance of symptoms.[54,55,56]

A study by Boris and Mandel found that dietary factors may play a significant role in the condition of the majority of children with ADHD. Of the children tested, 73% responded favourably to an elimination diet. The children reacted to various foods, dyes and preservatives.[57]

Breakey, in a 1997 review of key research, mainly from 1985-1995, on the relationship between food and behaviour concluded that the research has shown that diet definitely affects some children. But rather than becoming simpler the issue has become noticeably more complex. The range of suspect food items has broadened, and some non-food items are also implicated. Symptoms which may change include those seen in attention deficit disorder (ADD) and attention deficit hyperactivity disorder (ADHD), sleep problems and physical symptoms, with later research particularly emphasising changes in mood. The reports reviewed also show the range of individual differences both in the food substances producing reactions and in the areas of change.[58]

Kaplan et al conducted a ten week study in which all food was provided for the families of twenty four hyperactive preschool aged boys whose parents reported the existence of sleep problems or physical signs and symptoms. The diet used was far broader in scope than most that had been used in previous studies. It eliminated not only artificial colours and flavours but also chocolate, monosodium glutamate, preservatives, caffeine, and any substance that families reported might affect their child. The diet was also low in simple sugars, and, if the family reported a history of possible problems with cow's milk, it was dairy free. More than half of the boys showed improvement in behaviour and negligible placebo effects. In addition, several non-behavioural variables tended to improve including waking during the night and halitosis.[59]

A review of thirty five years of research on the links between diet and ADHD by Stevens et al concluded that there is a subgroup of children with ADHD who improve if artificial food colours are removed from their diet. Some children also seem to be sensitive to common non-salicylate foods such as milk, eggs, and wheat, as well as salicylate containing foods.[60]

In 2007, McCann et al published their findings on the links between food additives and hyperactive behaviour in children.[61] They had carried out a randomised double-blinded, placebo controlled trial to test whether the intake of artificial food colours and additives affected children's behaviour. The tests involved children in two age groups: three year olds, and eight to nine year olds.

They found that a mix of additives commonly found in children's food could exacerbate hyperactive behaviours such as inattention, impulsivity, and over-activity. Behavioural changes were noted in children who had been diagnosed with hyperactivity and also in children who had not. The additives used in this study were:

E102 Tartrazine, E104 Quinoline Yellow,
E110 Sunset Yellow, E122 Carmoisine,
E124 Ponceau 4R, E129 Allura Red
E211 Sodium Benzoate

At last there was a study that proved the link between behaviour and additives, and had been carried out in a way that was acceptable to the establishment. The editor of American Academy of Pediatrics Grand Rounds commented as follows: "The overall findings of the study are clear and require that even we skeptics who have long doubted parental claims of the effects of various foods on the behaviour of their children, admit we might have been wrong".[62]

It was quite strange watching official bodies and food manufacturers rushing to accommodate findings that literally weeks before they would have denied as being possible. In the UK food manufacturers began to make changes very quickly and the momentum increased so that from July 2010 a, European Union wide, warning has to be placed on any food or soft drink that contains any of the six colours—the label must carry the warning "may have adverse effects on activity and attention in children". Action in various other countries is also taking place to try implement similar measures.

See also *Behaviour*

Autism

A number of studies have reported a worsening of neurological symptoms in autistic individuals after the consumption of milk and wheat. Lucarelli et al tested the effectiveness of a cow's milk free diet, as well as some other foods, in thirty six autistic people. They noticed a marked improvement in the behavioural symptoms after eight weeks on an elimination diet and concluded that there is a link between food allergy and infantile autism.[63]

O'Banion et al studied the effect of particular foods on levels of hyperactivity, uncontrolled laughter, and disruptive behaviour in an eight-year old autistic boy. They found that, for this child, foods including wheat, corn, tomatoes, sugar, mushrooms, and dairy products produced behavioural disorders.[64]

Waring and Klovrza on examining the low plasma sulphate levels found in many autistic children state that "the most useful advice that can be given to parents of autistic children is to try a gluten-free, casein-free diet for at least 6 months, also removing chocolate, bananas and citrus fruit".[65] Reichelt found that for some autistic children diets that were either gluten-free and milk-reduced or milk-free and gluten-reduced resulted in an improvement in some behaviour problems and also a decrease in epileptic seizures.[66]

Hyperactivity is often a condition that occurs in children with autism spectrum disorder (ASD) which has led to some parents using variations of the Feingold diet. Srinivasan notes that "Salicylates are a subgroup of phenols, and some parents notice that patients with autism have occasional problems with breakdown of phenols".[67]

Behaviour

A survey of allergists in the US in 1950 found that more than half had noticed changes in personality when people known to have allergies were exposed to food triggers.[68]

Schauss reported that when several Michigan detention centres reduced their inmates' milk consumption, the incidence of antisocial behaviour also decreased.[69]

Crook, in 1980, reported on cases where dietary changes have had startling results in children. The examples he cites include aggressive behaviour being triggered by red dye, peanuts, wheat, sugar, and milk; hostile behaviour induced by milk; hyperactivity and irritability by red colours, citrus fruits, and potatoes.[70]

Swain et al found that eighty one out of a group of one hundred and forty children with behavioural disorders experienced significant improvement following the elimination of certain foods and food additives.[71] Novembre et al report on cases in which reactions to the food additives tartrazine and benzoate group led to a range of symptoms affecting the central nervous system including headaches, concentration and learning problems, depression and over activity.[72]

In a review paper, Hall notes that allergies of the nervous system have been found to cause diverse behavioural disturbances including headaches, convulsions, learning disabilities, schizophrenia and depression. Treatment includes using elimination and rotation diets. The observation is made that whilst some of the biological mechanisms have been established by research, others remain to be explored.[73]

In 1986, Vlissides et al carried out a double blind study on the effect of a gluten-free versus a gluten-containing diet in a ward of a maximum-security hospital. Most of the twenty four individuals suffered from psychotic disorders, particularly schizophrenia. Out of the twelve who had a gluten-free diet, two improved and relapsed when the gluten diet was reintroduced.[74]

See also *Attention Deficit Hyperactivity Disorder*

Breast Pain

A study in 1989 by Russell demonstrated a link between breast pain in women diagnosed with fibrocystic breast disease and caffeine intake. After the first year, 81.9% of the women involved had reduced their caffeine intake substantially and 61% of these reported a decrease or absence of breast pain.[75]

Chronic Fatigue Syndrome

In a paper, *Allergy and the chronic fatigue syndrome*, Straus concludes that allergies coexist with the chronic fatigue syndrome in more than 50% of people.[76]

In his book *Chronic Fatigue Syndrome* Dr Stoff outlines how food allergies and sensitivities are often a secondary problem that arises with CFS.[77]

There is also a great deal of anecdotal evidence of cases where individuals with debilitating CFS have had their symptoms reduced substantially, even eliminated, by a change in diet. Whether a cause or not, food sensitivities cannot be ignored by anyone suffering from CFS. Following general advice on a "healthy" diet will not be enough, sensitivities will need to be identified and accommodated in the diet.

See also *Fatigue*.

Coeliac Disease

Coeliac disease has been accepted as a condition that is usually triggered by ingestion of gluten in grains such as wheat and rye. The symptoms vary in type and severity from individual to individual but can include diarrhoea, excessive wind, and/or constipation, persistent or unexplained gastrointestinal symptoms, recurring stomach pain, cramping or bloating, tiredness, headaches, weight loss mouth ulcers, hair loss, skin rash, depression, tooth enamel problems, poor muscle co-ordination.[78]

There are various testing techniques available to identify if the individual does in fact have coeliac disease. If the condition is confirmed then lifelong adherence to a gluten-free diet is central to the treatment of this disease.[79]

See also *Colic and Colitis, Gastrointestinal Problems*

Colic and Colitis

Food allergy has been identified as one major cause of colitis in children which may become a lifelong problem leading to more serious conditions or resolve spontaneously.[80,81]

Hill et al studied the role of food allergies and problems with additives in babies suffering from colic and found a link between food problems and colic in 39% of the babies studied. They suggest that treatment of healthy babies with colic would usefully include a low allergen diet and appropriate nutritional support.[82]

Enterocolitis is an inflammation of the colon and small intestine. A study by Mehr et al examined various triggering factors including food for children with acute food protein-induced enterocolitis syndrome. Thirty five children experienced sixty six episodes of food protein-induced enterocolitis syndrome—vomiting was the most common symptom, followed by lethargy, pallor, and diarrhoea The majority reacted to a single food but six reacted to two foods. The problem foods were rice, soy, cow's milk, vegetables and fruits, oats, and fish. They concluded that "misdiagnosis and delays in diagnosis for children with food protein-induced enterocolitis syndrome were common, leading many children to undergo unnecessary, often painful investigations".[83]

See also *Coeliac Disease, Gastrointestinal Problems*

Crohn's Disease

Rudman et al maintained four people with Crohn's disease on a gluten-free and lactose-free diet for twelve days, after which they were challenge tested. Within four to nine days of beginning the gluten challenge they all developed reactions including fever, abdominal pain, diarrhoea, and nausea. The reactions subsided within two to four weeks after discontinuation of gluten.[84]

Jones et al was successful in inducing remission for some individuals with active Crohn's disease by dietary changes. The most frequent symptom-provoking foods were wheat, dairy products, brassicas (such as cabbage, broccoli, and cauliflower), corn, yeast, tomatoes, citrus fruits, and eggs.[85]

Dermatitis Herpetiformis

Dermatitis herpetiformis has frequently been linked with the consumption of foods containing gluten and, sometimes, dairy products. Atherton states that there can be no real doubt that dietary gluten is responsible for most, if not all, dermatitis herpetiformis.[86]

Various other studies have found similar links.[87,88,89] However, Kadunce et al found that dietary factors other than gluten were also important in the pathogenesis of the skin lesions in dermatitis herpetiformis.[90]

Eczema (and Dermatitis)

There are numerous studies linking eczema and dermatitis with food sensitivities. Atherton writes that foods appear to play an important provocative role in many instances of atopic eczema. The reaction often appears to be slow and insidious, is almost always unrecognised by the patient, and is not detected by skin testing or tests for IgE antibodies.[91]

Van Bever et al in a study of children with severe atopic dermatitis found the condition linked to reactions to eggs, wheat, milk, soya, and various additives including tartrazine, sodium benzoate, sodium glutamate and sodium metabisulphite.[92]

Soutter et al found that in sixty eight children with eczema, 79% had food allergies before the age of ten months and 23% at seven years of age.[93]

Burks et al linked atopic dermatitis to sensitivities to a range of foods including egg, milk, soya, wheat, cod/catfish, cashew and peanut.[94,95]

Sampson and McCaskill studied one hundred and thirteen children with severe atopic dermatitis and discovered that 56% had food sensitivities—egg, milk and peanut were the most common culprits.[96]

Hanifin in his study of the links between diet and atopic dermatitis suggests that between 10 and 20% of children and 10% of adults have eczema that is aggravated by food. The most common culprits being eggs, milk, peanuts, seafood, wheat and soya.[97]

Veien et al carried out a randomised, placebo-controlled oral challenge with preservatives and food colourings on one hundred and one individuals with eczema of undetermined origin but who suspected that the intake of certain foods aggravated their dermatitis. Thirty seven reacted to one or more of the food additives but not to a placebo.[98]

A six-year old boy's hands became red, swollen and painful. The cause was found to be lime juice. The boy's hands had been immersed in lime juice whilst he had been helping to make limeade.[99] A fifty-two year old woman had an eczematous rash at the side of her mouth and lips. The cause was discovered to be lime—she had been sucking the lime from her gin and tonic for up to 1 minute after finishing her drink.[100]

A seventy-eight year old woman experienced an extensive rash, diagnosed as dermatitis, all over her body including her face and scalp. The rash appeared two days after she had eaten a large amount of raw shitake mushrooms.[101]

Davies and Orton highlighted three cases of contact reactions to chapatti flour. One woman had a history of developing itchy weals on her hands immediately after handling chapatti flour. Prick testing to her chapatti flour as well as wheat flour and a scratch patch test to chapatti flour all produced positive weal and flare reactions. A thirty-six year old woman had a ten year history of hand eczema as well as sneezing within minutes of exposure to chapatti flour. Patch testing to her flour was negative, but scratch patch testing to chapatti flour and prick testing to wheat were both positive.

Another had a three year history of persistent hand eczema, affecting the palms of both hands and the fingertips. She experienced itching and burning of her hands immediately after handling chapatti flour. Skin prick tests to chapatti and wheat flour were both positive. These are all examples of contact reactions to the flour with none of the women reporting any symptoms after eating cooked chapatti.[102]

See also *Psoriasis, Urticaria.*

Epilepsy

There have been studies that have shown improvement or recovery from epileptic seizures as a result of ruling out food sensitivities. These were usually most marked in individuals who had additional symptoms such as migraines and digestive problems.

A study of children by Egger et al identified forty two different foods that caused seizures and symptoms in forty five children who had epilepsy with recurrent headaches, abdominal symptoms, or hyperkinetic behaviour. Thirty six of these recovered or improved when their problem foods were removed from their diets.[103]

Kinsman et al tried the ketogenic diet (high fat/low carbohydrate) with fifty eight epileptic children who required multiple medications. They found that seizure control improved in 67%, medication could be reduced in 64%, also greater dexterity and improved behaviour was noted in 36% and 23% respectively.[104]

Pelliccia et al explored the link between cow's milk allergy and epilepsy. Three children with cryptogenetic partial epilepsy and behavioural disorders such as hyperactivity and sleeping difficulties were placed on a milk-free diet. An improvement was observed in the children's behaviour and the electroencephalographic anomalies disappeared. Double blind oral provocation tests did not present an immediate reaction. Reactions occurred a few days after the test but, once placed on the diet again, they disappeared. They concluded that it was feasible that food intolerance could lead to the onset of convulsive crisis.[105]

Fatigue

Fatigue is a very common symptom of food intolerance but has rarely been studied in isolation as it is usually one of a number of symptoms.

Randolph and Moss present the case of a male college student with unexplained fatigue and other symptoms such as irritability and nervousness. After a food testing protocol was carried out, it was found that his fatigue was always brought on by dairy products and eggs. In another case the incriminating foods were pork, milk, egg, potatoes, beets and beet sugar.[106]

A Japanese study by Kondo et al showed how traditional methods of testing were not successful in identifying sensitivities to cow's milk and buckwheat in individuals with allergy-tension-fatigue yet these substances were the cause of their fatigue.[107]

See also *Chronic Fatigue Syndrome.*

Gallbladder Disease

Breneman conducted a study of sixty nine people with gallstones or post-cholecystectomy syndrome. They were all placed on elimination diets with foods being gradually reintroduced. All the people were relieved of their symptoms usually within three to five days. Egg was the most frequent offender (93%), followed by pork (64%) and onion (52%).[108]

Gastrointestinal Problems

Gastrointestinal symptoms including diarrhoea, nausea, abdominal cramping, and gastrointestinal bleeding are frequently associated with food sensitivity.[109] In a study of seventy one children with chronic abdominal pain, Ignys et al found that food allergies were implicated and that many improved after being placed on an elimination diet.[110]

Pelto et al hypothesised that milk hypersensitivity in adults may be the cause of gastrointestinal disorders. From the people they tested they did find a link that was not always associated with lactose intolerance and did not always show up as an actual allergy. They concluded that milk hypersensitivity in adults, occurring as gastrointestinal reactions, may be more common than previously thought.[111]

Read et al studied twenty seven people with severe chronic diarrhoea for which no diagnosis had previously been found. For one of the people the cause turned out to be an allergy to beef.[112] In a study of fifty people with ulcerative colitis, food allergy was found to be the cause in 67% of them.[113]

Rowe and Rowe reported that nearly 50% of one hundred and seventy people with ulcerative colitis needed no medication as their condition could be managed successfully with anti-allergy therapy alone.[114] Rider and Moeller tested twenty people with ulcerative colitis for wheat, egg and milk intolerance; fourteen of them experienced complete remission or significant improvement.[115]

Wright and Truelove placed fifty people with ulcerative colitis on a milk-free diet or a control diet for one year. During the follow-up period, 38% of those on the milk-free diet remained free of relapses, compared with 21% of those on the control diet.[116]

Food protein-induced enterocolitis syndrome (FPIES) in very young children leads to a range of symptoms including gastrointestinal distress, malabsorption, diarrhea, pain, and failure to thrive. Cow's milk and soya are the most common causes of FPIES, but cereal grains (rice, oat, and barley), fish, poultry, and vegetables can also cause the condition. In most cases, the problems have gone away by the time the child reaches the age of three.[117]

See also *Coeliac Disease, Colic and Colitis, Crohn's Disease, Irritable Bowel Syndrome.*

Glaucoma

In a review of the research, Mindell found that glaucoma can be caused by long term use of steroid drugs or by "over consumption of optic nerve toxins like aspartame and MSG (monosodium glutamate)".[118]

Head and Neck Pain

Seltzer reviewed the existing literature to uncover the existence of head and neck pain syndromes caused by foods, and food and drug combinations. They found at least twenty five such syndromes including those induced by colourings, flavours, chocolate, coffee and tea, and foods containing tyramine.[119]

Hemiplegia

Staffieri et al reported on a case of right sided hemiplegia that took place immediately after a meal. It was associated with angioedema, urticaria, purpura, and eosinophilia. A wheat elimination diet resulted in a clearance of the symptoms within a few days.[120]

Cooke reported on a case of transient third cranial nerve palsy associated with hemiparesis, followed by an episode of contralateral blindness and paresthesia in a food allergic patient. Symptoms were resolved with avoidance of beef and pork.[121]

Hypoglycaemia

Blood sugar problems are usually linked with diets that are high in refined carbohydrates such as white bread and sugar. The advice is to avoid refined carbohydrates and to switch to a high carbohydrate/high fibre diet or a high protein/low carbohydrate diet. However, for many people neither of these will work as their blood sugar problems are caused by a food sensitivity. Breneman identified food sensitivities as the cause of blood sugar problems in 75% of those with the condition.[122]

Irritable Bowel Syndrome (IBS)

Petitpierre, Gumowski, and Girard investigated food hypersensitivity as a cause of irritable bowel syndrome. They found that one or several foods or food additives could induce the typical symptoms of IBS and that adequate exclusion diets could result in dramatic clinical improvements.[123]

Nanda et al had people with irritable bowel syndrome placed on an elimination diet for three weeks. The diet excluded dairy products, cereals, citrus fruits, potatoes, tea, coffee, alcohol, additives, and preservatives. Improvement was experienced by 42.8%. Some were intolerant of only one food and others had multiple food intolerances, the maximum being nineteen. The most common problem foods were dairy products, onions, wheat, chocolate, coffee, eggs, nuts, citrus fruits, tea, rye, potatoes, barley, oats, and corn.[124]

Antico et al concluded that food additives may be a major factor in the development of irritable bowel syndrome.[125]

Joint Pain

In cases studied by Novembre et al, tartrazine and benzoates were linked with causing joint pain.[126] Golding reported that nine individual's attacks of joint pain and associated swelling were triggered by certain foods or associated with allergic manifestations.[127]

A naturopath and orthomolecular nutritionist, Alexander writes that he has found "70 per cent of the people he treats for joint pain and stiffness and/or muscle pain have a sensitivity to the nightshade group of plants". His experience led him to write that an "important part of the treatment of arthritis is the removal of this food group from the diet".[128]

Solanine is a naturally occurring chemical that is found in these plants and is dealt with in a later section.

See also *Arthritis*.

Mekersson-Rosenthal Syndrome

Food allergy and intolerance to food additives have been implicated in Mekersson-Rosenthal syndrome. Mckenna et al report on the case of a thirty-four year old man whose symptoms were triggered by sodium benzoate and tartrazine.[129]

Memory Loss

Impaired memory is a not uncommon symptom of food intolerance but it is rarely one that is studied in isolation as it invariably comes in tangent with other symptoms. Randolph and Moss present the case of a woman who had an excellent memory and then began to experience memory loss. Initially her problem was thought to be psychological in origin but was found to be caused by a susceptibility to wheat, corn and, especially, oats.[130]

Dr Mandell refers to a condition known as "allergic amnesia" in which the allergy sufferer often lashes out verbally, has irrational outbursts, and may be aggressive but later has no memory of the incident. He also cites cases of memory loss caused by food intolerance: one of a woman with periodic memory lapses, the other of a boy who after eating chocolate suffered from an impaired memory.[131]

Meniere's Disease

Derebery and Berliner found that 40.3% of seven hundred and thirty four people with Meniere's disease had or suspected they had food allergies.[132] In a different study, Derebery concluded that people with Meniere's disease can show improvement in their symptoms of tinnitus and vertigo when receiving specific allergy therapy.[133]

Haid et al in a study of five hundred and seventy four individuals suffering from Meniere's disease found that, amongst other factors, allergy may trigger the disease.[134]

Migraine

Migraines have over the years been linked with a wide range of foods. Some studies also link them with naturally occurring food chemicals such as histamine and tyramine.

Food allergy as a cause of migraine is mentioned in the scientific literature as early as 1930 when Blayeat and Brittain published the results of their study of fifty five migraine sufferers. In that study, 52.7% achieved complete or near-complete freedom from symptoms by avoiding allergenic foods; a further 38.2% had some degree of partial improvement.[135]

Speer found that foods such as milk, chocolate, cola and corn, were common triggers for migraine.[136] A study by Grant of sixty people with a history, some as long as twenty two years, of frequent and recurring migraines had 85% of them become headache-free after following an elimination diet. The number of headaches in the group fell from four hundred and two to only six per month. The commonest foods causing reactions were wheat (78%), orange (65%), eggs (45%), tea and coffee (40% each), chocolate and milk (37% each), beef (35%), corn, cane sugar, and yeast (33% each).[137]

Scheife and Hills found that amongst the most common precipitating factors for migraine were foods and drinks including coffee, tea, and cola beverages, chocolate, cheese, and alcohol.[138]

Merret et al tested to see if food allergy was a major cause of migraine. Their findings were that allergies could not often be detected and concluded that the food intolerance associated with migraine headaches was not related to the conventionally defined allergic mechanism.[139] Mansfield noted that clinical observations and studies support the role of food in causing migraine and sinus headache and clearly makes the point that the benefits of an avoidance diet include the need for fewer medications.[140]

Lucarelli et al studied ninety two children affected by migraine. Forty nine had positive skin tests to one or more foods and forty of these improved after following an elimination diet for four to six weeks.[141] Elimination diets worked for migraine sufferers in a study by Mylek. The food most usually implicated was cow's milk but other problem foods included cabbage, eggs, preservatives and colours, some cheeses, and chocolate.[142]

A study by Wantke using a histamine free diet had considerable success for some migraine sufferers.[143] Leira and Rodriguez reported that some foods in our diet can spark off migraine attacks in susceptible individuals. They identified a number of food based triggers for migraine including individual foods such as cheese, citrus fruits, nuts, tea, coffee, pork, chocolate, milk, vegetables, and substances within food such as tyramine, phenylalanine, phenolic flavonoids, alcohol, caffeine, food additives including sodium nitrate, monosodium glutamate and aspartame.[144]

Mouth Ulcers (Aphthous Ulcers)

Wray reports on a study in which twenty individuals who had suffered from recurrent aphthous ulcers, some for more than eleven years, were given a gluten-free diet to follow. Five (25%) became ulcer free and when challenge tested with gluten the ulcers returned.[145]

A study by Hay and Reade placed seventeen individuals with recurrent aphthous ulcers that had not responded to conventional therapy on an elimination diet. Of the twelve people who followed the diet for six to eight weeks, four became symptom-free and one had marked improvement. In four of these cases a particular food was identified which, when eliminated from the diet, led to marked improvement or complete resolution of the ulcers.[146] Similar results were found by Wright et al.[147]

Movement Disorders

Gerrard et al present three cases where individuals had episodic movement disorders triggered by foods or components of the diet. In one person, the movement consisted of shaking the head from side to side and was triggered by milk and a number of other foods. Repeated shrugging of the shoulders, in another, was triggered by egg and coffee. Rhythmic contractions of the arms and legs, in the third individual, were triggered by aspartame. Their observations led the researchers to conclude that foods can trigger movement disorder by acting on dopamine and other neurotransmitter pathways in the brain.[148]

Multiple Sclerosis

Dr Mandell describes the case of a woman who had been diagnosed with multiple sclerosis. After extensive allergy testing it was found that most of her symptoms were in fact caused by food sensitivities.[149]

Murray and Pizzorno note that "the consumption of two common allergens—gluten and milk—have been implicated in MS".[150]

Kruger and Nyland have proposed that "multiple sclerosis arises due to the effect of various mediators (histamine and protease) released from the perivascular mast cells after stimulation by some diet factor."[151]

Nephrotic Syndrome

Nephrotic syndrome is a condition marked by very high levels of protein in the urine, low levels of protein in the blood, swelling especially around the eyes, feet, and hands, and high cholesterol. It can occur with many diseases but some causes are unknown. The following studies all demonstrate how in some of these cases the problem can be food intolerance.

Sandberg et al studied six children, aged between ten and thirteen, who all had nephrotic syndrome of unknown origin. Drug treatment was stopped and a diet that avoided milk was prescribed. Once the protein in the urine had dropped to a certain level, within three to ten days, the children were challenge tested with milk. The milk challenge resulted in a return of significant amounts of protein in the urine and oedema in four of the children.[152]

Gaboardi et al outlined the case of a six-year old girl with dermatitis herpetiformis, coeliac disease, and nephrotic syndrome. All three conditions disappeared when she was placed on a gluten-free diet.[153]

Lagrue et al tested thirty four individuals with idiopathic nephrotic syndrome. Five foods were tested—wheat flour, cow's milk, whole egg, beef and pork. The tests were positive in twenty two of the individuals.[154] Various other studies have confirmed that for some individuals there is a link between food sensitivies and idiopathic nephrotic syndrome. [155,156,157,158,159]

Oral Allergy Syndrome

Oral allergy syndrome refers to symptoms that arise as a result of direct contact of the oral mucosa with the offending food. Symptoms are usually in the form of oral itching and lip swelling. It has been frequently associated with sensitisation to fresh fruits and vegetables in those with a pollen allergy. Bircher et al found that about 35% of people allergic to pollens showed allergic symptoms to fresh fruit and vegetables.[160]

Oral allergy syndrome has also been described in cases of egg and shrimp allergy.[161] Adults seem to be more likely to develop oral allergy syndrome to fresh fruit and vegetables than children.

Pre Menstrual Syndrome

Although it is unlikely that PMS is as such "caused" by food intolerance, reactions to problem foods can be exacerbated in the pre-menstrual phase and may mimic PMS symptoms. Abraham found that symptoms of the pre-menstrual syndrome could be reduced or eliminated by changes in the diet—either by eliminating/reducing certain foods or increasing supplementation of certain vitamins.[162,163]

Wurtman et al found an association between changes in mood and eating carbohydrates. They found that women who reported having pre-menstrual symptoms increased their intake of carbohydrates when feeling depressed. They speculate that this is an attempt to increase serotonin production and hence improve mood.[164] It seems possible that certain foods will "agree" or "aggravate" more at certain times in the menstrual cycle.

Psoriasis

Skin conditions are frequently linked with contact or food sensitivities and psoriasis is no exception. Douglas reported on people with psoriasis improving after eliminating certain foods. The foods varied from individual to individual but included citrus fruits, nuts, corn and milk. Others noticed improvement when eating a diet low in acidic foods such as coffee, tomatoes, soda and pineapple.[165]

Michaelsson et al found that a gluten-free diet was helpful to some people with psoriasis.[166]

See also *Eczema, Urticaria*.

Recurrent Otitis Media

Inflammation of the middle ear is a common childhood complaint. In 1994, Nsouli et al evaluated one hundred and four children, with recurrent serious otitis media, for food allergy by means of skin testing, specific IgE tests, and food challenges. Children who had evidence of allergy eliminated the suspected offending foods for sixteen weeks, after which individual food challenges were done.

Eighty one (78%) of the children had evidence of food allergy, and elimination of the allergens resulted in significant improvement in 86 percent of the children. The problem foods were cow's milk, wheat, egg white, peanut, soya, corn, orange, chicken and apple. They concluded that considering food allergies in children with these problems "might prevent surgery and might prevent permanent damage".[167]

Viscomi presents an approach to allergic management for use in cases of children with otitis media arguing that there is often a history of allergy. Fifty allergic children with recurrent secretory otitis media, despite conventional surgical therapy, were treated for inhalant and food allergy for one year. There was a significant reduction in the recurrence of the condition.[168]

A study by Bernstein et al of 100 children with recurrent otitis media with effusion tested for six inhalant and two food allergens. They concluded that allergic reactions may play a role in otitis media with effusion in about 23% of young allergic patients. One wonders if the percentage would have been significantly higher if a greater range of foods had been tested.[169]

Rousquet et al reported that between 7 and 29% of asthma sufferers have a milk sensitivity. They also found it was often a cause of rhinoconjuctivitis in young children and may be implicated in serious otitis media.[170]

Restless Legs Syndrome

In a study of people with restless legs syndrome, Lutz found many improved on a caffeine free diet.[171]

Rhinitis

Rhinitis is a symptom usually associated with hay fever but studies, including those carried out by Pelikan,[172] Pastorello,[173] and Freedman,[174] have shown that when food, including additives, are tested there is a surprisingly high number of patients who have some degree of intolerance, sensitivity or allergy.

Sampson and Eigenmann estimate that the prevalence of food-induced allergic rhinitis, even among patients referred to allergy clinics, appears to be less than 1 percent, although 25 to 80 percent of patients with documented IgE-mediated food allergy have nasal symptoms during oral food challenges.[175] Cinqi et al note that food-induced allergic rhinitis frequently occurs together with other food allergy symptoms such as asthma, eczema, oral allergic manifestations, urticaria, and gastrointestinal symptoms.[176]

Kok et al involved six hundred and eighty individuals who were receiving treatment for allergic rhinitis in a study in which they were tested for various food allergies. Common positive foods were tested, including hidden ingredient foods such as soy, wheat and malt. Twenty one per cent reported poor to slight improvement, 29.4% reported better improvement, and nearly 50% reported good to very good improvement. Three of the most common allergens were egg, milk, and wheat. The study authors concluded that strict diet control without pharmacotherapy is effective in the management of patients with food-induced allergic rhinitis.[177]

Raphael et al explores "gustatory rhinitis", a form of rhinorrhea caused by spicy foods in which the reactions are not immunological ones, being influenced rather by neurologic mechanisms.[178]

Sexual Dysfunction

Armani et al had seven young men eat seven grams of liquorice each day for a week, They found that after four days their testosterone levels had dropped by an average of 44%. These findings led them to suggest that doctors should consider liquorice as a potential culprit when treating men with sexual dysfunction.[179]

Sinusitis

Allergy was demonstrated to be an underlying factor in 40 to 67% of people with chronic sinusitis and is present in as many as 80% of people with bilateral sinusitis according to Spector.[180]

Mansfield noted that clinical observations and studies support the role of food in causing migraine and sinus headache and clearly makes the point that the benefits of an avoidance diet include the need for fewer medications.[181]

Sleep Disorders

Okudaira et al found that ingestion of xanthines such as theophylline and caffeine in coffee, tea, colas, and chocolate could contribute to some sleep disorders.[182]

Kahn et al in a study of one hundred and forty six children referred for sleep disturbance identified fifteen whose sleep problems were resolved within five weeks of starting a diet free from cow's milk. In a subsequent challenge, the sleep disturbances returned within four days of reintroducing the cow's milk.[183] Food chemicals, such as salicylate, have also been implicated in sleep disturbances.

Tinnitus

Tinnitus is an accepted symptom of salicylate toxicity as has been frequently shown in various studies. For example, Brien's review of toxicity associated with salicylates cites tinnitus and hearing loss, usually reversible, with acute intoxication and long term administration of salicylates such as aspirin.[184]

And, Cazals notes that tinnitus may be the first subjectively recognised symptom of salicylate toxicity and presents evidence going back to 1877 which shows links between salicylates and tinnitus. The dose of salicylate medications, for the treatment of rheumatoid arthritis, was often set below the point at which the individual started to experience tinnitus.[185]

Although these studies have focused on manufactured forms of salicylate there is also evidence that dietary salicylate, in a sensitive individual, may also lead to tinnitus. DeBartolo reported that over a twelve year period they had identified individuals who were sensitive to salicylates and had improved or relieved their tinnitus with a salicylate free diet.[186] Shulman in his book on the diagnosis and treatment of tinnitus includes one of the potential triggers as being foods high in salicylate.

Urticaria

Atherton writes that food has been demonstrated to play a major role in urticaria. In some people whealing occurs within minutes of ingestion of the problem food, in others the reaction can be much slower and less easy to identify. It is not only foods that cause these reactions but food additives, especially azo dyes, have been implicated.[187]

Swain et al found that eighty six out of one hundred and forty children with recurrent urticaria improved significantly on a salicylate free diet. They also observed reactions to preservatives, azo dyes and brewer's yeast.[188] Juhlin also found that many sufferers of urticaria improved on a diet free from additives.[189]

Henz and Zuberbier reported that in the majority of cases of urticaria the symptoms were provoked, and sustained, by food ingredients. On a diet largely avoiding preservatives, dyes and natural pseudo allergens, 73% of people experienced remission of more than six months duration, starting within the first three weeks after starting the diet (the spontaneous remission rate is 14%). Eighteen per cent reacted to food preservatives and dyes, and 71% to pureed tomatoes.[190]

Zuberbier et al had success in identifying food additives as the cause of urticaria in some people and improvement in the symptoms of others.[191] Verschave et al used an elimination diet for additives and tyramine with sixty seven individuals with chronic urticaria; 55% reacted favourably.[192] Rudzki et al placed one hundred and fifty eight people with chronic urticaria on a diet free of salicylates, benzoates and azo dyes—fifty were found to be sensitive to food additives.[193]

Thirty per cent of individuals with chronic urticaria and angioneurotic oedema, in a study by Montano et al, were found to be sensitive to sodium benzoate, tartrazine or sodium metabisulfite.[194]

See also *Eczema, Psoriasis.*

Vasculitis

Veien and Krogdahl reported on the case of a twenty-four year old woman with leukocytoclastic vasculitis. She experienced a severe eruption of vasculitis after a placebo controlled oral challenge with 50mg of ponceau (E214, a red colour dye). She followed an additive free diet and, after two months, the vasculitis was found to have faded.[195]

Buscino et al described the cases of two children with food induced vasculitis. In an eight-year old girl, the vasculitis was found to be caused by a sensitivity to cow's milk and also to eggs. A twenty-three month old girl with vasculitis was found to be sensitive to chocolate: the vasculitis went into remission when chocolate was avoided and only returned after accidental ingestion of products containing cocoa.[196]

Vertigo

Dunn and Snyder presented information on three children who were found to be milk sensitive. Their vertigo attacks were eliminated by removing milk from their diets and reappeared with milk challenges. Chocolate was suspected in another child but could not be confirmed.[197] Duke reported on a case of adult vertigo in Meniere's syndrome that improved on an elimination diet.[198]

References

[1] Mackarness R. Not All In The Mind. Pan 1976.

[2] Coca AF. Familial Nonreaginic Food Allergy. Charles C Thomas 1945.

[3] Mandell M, Scanlon L W. Dr Mandell's 5-Day Allergy Relief System. Thomas Y Crowell 1979.

[4] Joneja JV. Dietary Management of Food Allergies and Intolerances: A Comprehensive Guide. Second edition. J.A. Hall Publications, 1998.

[5] Rinkel H J, Randolph TG, Zeller M. Food Allergy. Thomas 1951.

[6] Mumby K. Food Allergies and Environmental Illness: the complete guide to. 1993 Thorsons.

[7] Speer G. Allergy of the Nervous System. Thomas 1970.

[8] Hare, Francis. The Food Factor in Disease. London: Longmans, Vol. I, II, 1905.

[9] Randolph TG, Moss R W. An Alternative Approach to Allergies: The new field of clinical ecology unravels the environmental causes of mental and physical ills (revised edition). Perennial Library, Harper & Row 1990.

[10] Philpott W H, Kalita D H. Brain Allergies: The Psychonutrient and Magnetic Connections. Keats 2000.

[11] Martin P. The Sickening Mind: Brain Behaviour, Immunity and Disease. Harper Collins 1997.

[12] Philpott W H, Kalita D H. Brain Allergies: The Psychonutrient and Magnetic Connections. Keats 2000.

[13] Rapaport HG. The Complete Allergy Guide. Simon and Schuster, 1970.

[14] Rea WJ, Peters DW, Smiley RE, Edgar R, Greenberg M, Fenyves E. Recurrent environmentally triggered thrombophlebitis: a five year follow-up. Ann Allergy 1981;(5Pt1):338-44.

[15] Vickers A, Zollman C. ABC of complementary medicine: Unconventional approaches to nutritional medicine. BMJ 1999;319:1419-1422.

[16] Mansfield J. Arthritis, Allergy, Nutrition and the Environment. Thorsons 1995

[17] http://www.allergyresearchfoundation.org/More-Allergy-Facts/ Jan, 2012.

[18] Gupta R, Sheikh A, Strachan DP, Anderson HR (2006) Time trends in allergic disorders in the UK. Thorax,. doi: 10.1136/thx.2004.038844

[19] http://news.bbc.co.uk/1/hi/health/440610.stm

[20] Moneret-Vautrin DA et al. The multifood allergy syndrome. Allerg Immunol (Paris) 2000;32(1):12-5.

[21] http://www.cdc.gov/nchs/data/databriefs/db10.htm

[22] Mumby K. Food Allergies and Environmental Illness: the complete guide to. 1993 Thorsons.

[23] Matteo A, Sarles H. Is food allergy a cause of acute pancreatitis? Pancreas 1990 Mar;5(2):234-7.

[24] de Diego Lorenzo A, Robles Fornieles J, Herrero Lopez T, Cos Arregui E. Acute pancreatitis associated with milk allergy. Int J Pancreatol 1992 Dec;12(3):319-21.

[25] Gastaminza G, Bernaola G, Camino ME. Acute pancreatitis caused by allergy to kiwi fruit. Allergy 1998 Nov;53(11):1104-5.

[26] Stolze I, Peters KP, Herbst RA. Histamine intolerance mimics anorexia nervosa. Hautarzt 2010 Sep;61(9):776-778.

[27] Mansfield J. Arthritis, Allergy, Nutrition and the Environment. Thorsons 1995.

[28] Hicklin JA, McEwen LM, Morgan JE. The effect of diet in rheumatoid arthritis. Clin Allergy 1980;10:463.

[29] Ratner D, Eshel E, Schneeyour A, Teitler A. Does milk intolerance affect seronegative arthritis in lactase-deficient women? Isr J Med Sci 1985;21:532-534.

[30] Panush RS, Stroud RM, Webster EM. Food-induced (allergic) arthritis. Inflammatory arthritis exacerbated by milk. Arthritis Rheum 1986;29(2):220-6.

[31] Beri D, Malaviya AN, Shandilya R, Singh RR. Effect of dietary restrictions on disease activity in rheumatoid arthritis. Ann Rheum Dis 1988;47:69-72.

[32] Darlington LG. Dietary therapy for arthritis. Rheum Dis Clin North Am 1991;7:273-285.

[33] Businco L, Falconieri P, Giampietro P, Bellioni B. Food allergy and asthma. Pediatr Pulmonol Suppl 1995;11:59-60.

[34] Stevenson DD, Simon RA. Sensitivity to ingested metabisulfites in asthmatic subjects. J Allergy Clin Immunol 1981;68:26-32.

[35] Stenius BSM, Lemola M. Hypersensitivity to acetylsalicylic acid (ASA) and tartrazine in patients with asthma. Clin Allergy 1976;6:119-129.

[36] Freedman BJ. Asthma induced by sulphur dioxide, benzoate and tartrazine contained in orange drinks. Clin Allergy 1977;7:407-415.

[37] Pelikan Z, Pelikan-Filipek M. Bronchial response to the food ingestion challenge. Ann Allergy 1987;58:164-172.

[38] Allen DH, Delohery J, Baker G. Monosodium L-glutamate-induced asthma. J Allergy Clin Immunol 1987;80(4):530-7.

[39] Eriksson NE. Food sensitivity reported by patients with asthma and hay fever. A relationship between food sensitivity and birch pollen-allergy

and between food sensitivity and acetylsalicylic acid intolerance. Allergy 1978;33(4):189-96.

[40] Rousquet J, Chanez P, Michel F-B. The respiratory tract and food hypersensitivity. In: Metcalfe DD, Sampson HA, Simon RA. (eds) Food Allergy: Adverse reactions to foods and food additives, 2nd ed. Blackwell Science 1997.

[41] Genton C, Frei PC, Pecoud A. Value of oral provocation tests to aspirin and food additives in the routine investigation of asthma and chronic urticaria. J Allergy Clin Immunol 1985;76(1):40-5.

[42] Pirson F, Detry B, Pilette C.Occupational rhinoconjuctivitis and asthma caused by chicory and oral allergy syndrome associated with bet v 1-related protein. J Investig Allergol Clin Immunol. 2009;19(4):306-10

[43] Kidd PM. Attention Deficit/Hyperactivity Disorder (ADHD) in Children: Rationale for Its Integrative Management Altern Med Rev 2000;5(5):402-428.

[44] Feingold B. Why your child is hyperactive. Random House 1985.

[45] Shannon WR. Neuropathic manifestations in infants and children as a result of anaphylactic reactions to foods contained in their diet. Am J Child Dis 1922;24:89-94.

[46] Schardt D. Diet and behavior in children. Nutrition Action Healthletter 2000;27:10-11. Washington, DC: Center for Science in the Public Interest.

[47] Kidd PM. Attention Deficit/Hyperactivity Disorder (ADHD) in Children: Rationale for Its Integrative Management Altern Med Rev 2000;5(5):402-428.

[48] Boris M. Food and chemical intolerance: Placebo-controlled studies in attention deficit disorders. In: Bellanti JA, Crook WG, Layton RE, eds. Attention Deficit Hyperactivity Disorder: Causes and Possible Solutions (Proceedings of a Conference). Jackson, TN: International Health Foundation; 1999.

[49] Boris M. Food and chemical intolerance: Placebo-controlled studies in attention deficit disorders. In: Bellanti JA, Crook WG, Layton RE, eds. Attention Deficit Hyperactivity Disorder: Causes and Possible Solutions (Proceedings of a Conference). Jackson, TN: International Health Foundation; 1999.

[50] Boris M, Mandel FS. Foods and additives are common causes of the attention deficit hyperactive disorder in children. Ann Allergy 1994;72:462-468.

[51] Murray MT, Pizzorno JT. Encyclopaedia of Natural Medicine. Rocklin, CA: Prima Publishing; 1998.

[52] Carter CM, Urbanowicz M, Hemsley R, Mantilla L, Strobel S, Graham PJ, Taylor E. Effects of a few food diet in attention deficit disorder. Arch Dis Child 1993;69(5):564-8.

[53] Crook WG. Sugar, yeast and ADHD: fact or fiction? In: Bellanti JA, Crook WG, Layton RE, eds. Attention Deficit Hyperactivity Disorder: Causes and Possible Solutions (Proceedings of a Conference). Jackson, TN: International Health Foundation; 1999.

[54] Egger J, Carter CM, Graham PJ, et al. Controlled trial of oligoantigenic treatment in the hyperkinetic syndrome. Lancet 1985;i:540-545.

[55] Egger J, Stolla A, McEwen LM, et al. Controlled trial of hyposensitisation in children with food-induced hyperkinetic syndrome. Lancet 1992;339:1150-1153.

[56] Swain A, Soutter V, Loblay R, et al. Salicylates, oligoantigenic diets, and behaviour. Lancet 1985;2 :41-42

[57] Boris M, Mandel FS. Foods and additives are common causes of the attention deficit hyperactive disorder in children. Ann Allergy 1994;72:462-468.

[58] Breakey J. The role of diet and behaviour in childhood. J Paediatr Child Health 1997;33(3):190-4.

[59] Kaplan BJ, McNicol J, Conte RA, Moghadam HK. Dietary replacement in preschool-aged hyperactive boys. Pediatrics 1989;83(1):7-17.

[60] Stevens LJ, Kuczek T, Burgess JR, Hurt E, Arnold LE. Dietary sensitivities and ADHD symptoms: thirty-five years of research. Clin Pediatr (Phila). 2011 Apr;50(4):279-93.

[61] McCann D, Barrett A, Cooper A, Crumpler D, Dalen L, Grimshaw K, Kitchin E, et al. Food additives and hyperactive behaviour in 3-year-old and 8/9-year-old children in the community: a randomised, double-blinded, placebo-controlled trial. Lancet. 2007 Nov 3;370(9598):1560-7.

[62] Editor. ADHD and Food Additives revisited. AAP Grand Rounds. 2008; 19:17.

[63] Lucarelli S, Frediani T, Zingoni AM, Ferruzzi F, Giardini O, Quintieri F, Barbato M, D'Eufemia P, Cardi E. Food allergy and infantile autism. Panminerva Med 1995;37(3):137-41.

[64] O'Banion D, Armstrong B, Cummings RA, Stange J. Disruptive behavior: a dietary approach. J Autism Child Schiz 1978 ;8(3):325-37.

[65] Waring RH, Klovrza LV. Sulphur Metabolism in Autism. J Nut Env Med 2000;10:25-32.

[66] Reichelt R. Gluten, Milk Proteins and Autism: Dietary Intervention Effects on Behaviour and Peptide Secretion. J App Nutr 1990;42(1).

[67] Srinivasan, P. A Review of dietary interventions in autism. Ann. Clin. Psych. 21:4, Nov. 2009, 237-247.

[68] Clarke TW. The relation of allergy to character problems in children; A survey. Ann Allergy 1950;8:75-87.

[69] Schauss AG. Nutrition and antisocial behaviour. Int Clin Nutr Review 1984;4(4):172-7.

[70] Crook WG. Can what a child eats make him dull, stupid or hyperactive? J Learn Dis, 1980;13:53-8.

[71] Swain A, Soutter V, Loblay R, et al. Salicylates, oligoantigenic diets, and behaviour. Lancet 1985;2 :41-42.

[72] Novembre E, Dini L, Bernardini R, Resti M, Vierucci A . Unusual reactions to food additives. Pediatr Med Chir 1992;14(1): 39-42.

[73] Hall K. Allergy of the nervous system: a review. Ann Allergy 1976;36(1):49-64.

[74] Vlissides DN, Venulet A, Jenner FA 2. A double-blind gluten-free/gluten-load controlled trial in a secure ward population. Br J Psychiatry 1986;148:447-5.

[75] Russell L C. Caffeine restriction as initial treatment for breast pain. Nurse Pract 1989;14(2):36-37,40.

[76] Straus SE, Dale JK, Wright R, Metcalfe DD. Allergy and the chronic fatigue syndrome. J Allergy Clin Immunol 1988; 81(5 Pt 1):791-5.

[77] Stoff J A, Pellegrino CR. Chronic fatigue Syndrome: The Hidden epidemic. Harper-Collins 1992.

[78] http://www.coeliac.org.uk/coeliac-disease/what-is-coeliac-disease

[79] Scanlon SA, Murray JA. Update on celiac disease - etiology, differential diagnosis, drug targets, and management advances. Clin Exp Gastroenterol. 2011;4:297-311.

[80] Hill SM et al. Colitis caused by food allergy in infants. Archives of Disease in Childhood 1990;65:1.

[81] Jenkins HR, Pincott JR, Soothill JF, Milla PJ, Harries JT. Food allergy: the major cause of infantile colitis. Arch Dis Child 1984 Apr;59(4):326-9.

[82] Hill SM et al. Colitis caused by food allergy in infants. Archives of Disease in Childhood 1990;65:1.

[83] Mehr S, Kakakios A, Frith K, Kemp AS. Food protein-induced enterocolitis syndrome: 16-year experience. Pediatrics. 2009 Mar;123(3):e459-64.

[84] Rudman D, Galambos JT, Wenger J, Achord JL. Adverse effects of dietary gluten in four patients with regional enteritis. Am J Clin Nutr 1971;24:1068-1073.

[85] Jones VA, Dickinson RJ, Workman E, Wilson AJ, Freeman AH, Hunter JO. Crohn's disease: maintenance of remission by diet. Lancet 1985,27;2(8448):177-80.

[86] Atherton DJ. Diagnosis and management of skin disorders caused by food allergy. Ann Allergy 1984;53(6Pt2):623-8.

[87] Garioch JJ, Lewis HM, Sargent SA, Leonard JN, Fry L. 25 years' experience of a gluten-free diet in the treatment of dermatitis herpetiformis. Br J Dermatol 1994;131(4):541-5.

[88] Fry L. Dermatitis herpetiformis. Baillieres Clin Gastroenterol 1995; 9(2):371-93.

[89] Gawkrodger DJ, Blackwell JN, Gilmour HM, Rifkind EA, Heading RC, Barnetson RS. Dermatitis herpetiformis: diagnosis, diet and demography. Gut, 1984;25(2):151-7.

[90] Kadunce DP, McMurry MP, Avots-Avotins A, Chandler JP, Meyer LJ, Zone JJ. The effect of an elemental diet with and without gluten on disease activity in dermatitis herpetiformis. J Invest Dermatol 1991;97(2):175-82.

[91] Atherton DJ. Diagnosis and management of skin disorders caused by food allergy. Ann Allergy 1984;53(6Pt2):623-8.

[92] Van Bever HP, Docx M, Stevens WJ. Food and food additives in severe atopic dermatitis. Allergy 1989;44(8):588-94.

[93] Soutter V, Swain A, Loblay, R. Food allergy and food intolerance in young children. Asia Pacific Journal of Clinical Nutrition 1995;4(3):329.

[94] Burks AW, James JM, Hiegel A, Wilson G, Wheeler JG, Jones SM, Zuerlein N. Atopic dermatitis and food hypersensitivity reactions. J Pediatr 1998;132(1):132-6.

[95] Burks AW, Mallory SB, Williams LW, Shirrell MA. Atopic dermatitis: clinical relevance of food hypersensitivity reactions. J Pediatr 1988;113(3):447-51.

[96] Sampson HA, McCaskill CC. Food hypersensitivity and atopic dermatitis: evaluation of 113 patients. J Pediatr 1985;107(5):669-75.

[97] Hanifin J M et al. Diet and atopic dermatitis. Western J of Med 1989;151:6.

[98] Veien NK, Hattel T, Justesen O, Norholm A. Oral challenge with food additives. Contact Dermatitis 1987;17(2):100-3.

[99] Wagner AM, Wu JJ, Hansen RC, Nigg HN, Beiere RC. Bullous phytophotodermatitis associated with high natural concentrations of furanocoumarins in limes. Am J Contact Dermat. 2002 Mar;13(1):10-4.

[100] Thomson MA, Preston PW, Prais L, Foulds IS. Lime dermatitis from gin and tonic with a twist of lime. Contact Dermatitis. 2007 Feb;56(2):114-5.

[101] Herault M, Waton J, Bursztejn AC, Schmutz JL, Barbaud A. Shiitake dermatitis now occurs in France. Ann Dermatol Venereol 2010 Apr;137(4):290-293.

[102] Davies E, Orton D. Contact urticaria and protein contact dermatitis to chapatti flour. Contact Dermatitis 2009 Feb;60(2):113-114.

[103] Egger J, Carter CM, Soothill JF, Wilson J. Oligoantigenic diet treatment of children with epilepsy and migraine. J Pediatr 114: 51-58, 1989.

[104] Kinsman SL, Vining EPG, Quaskey SA, Mellitis D, Freeman JM. Efficacy of the ketogenic diet for intractable seizure disorders: review of 58 cases. Epilepsia 1992;33:1132-36.

[105] Pelliccia A, Lucarelli S, Frediani T, D'Ambrini G, Cerminara C, Barbato M, Vagnucci B, Cardi E. Partial cryptogenetic epilepsy and food allergy/intolerance. A causal or a chance relationship? Reflections on three clinical cases. Minerva Pediatr 1999;51(5):153-7.

[106] Randolph TG, Moss R W. An Alternative Approach to Allergies: The new field of clinical ecology unravels the environmental causes of mental and physical ills (revised edition). Perennial Library, Harper & Row 1990.

[107] Kondo N, Shinoda S, Agata H, Nishida T, Miwa Y, Fujii H, Orii T. Lymphocyte responses to food antigens in food sensitive patients with allergic tension-fatigue syndrome. Biotherapy 1992;5(4):281-4.

[108] Breneman J. Allergy elimination diet as the most effective gall bladder diet. Ann Allergy 1968;26:83.

[109] James JM, Burks AW. Food-associated gastrointestinal disease. Curr Opin Pediatr 1996;8(5):471-5.

[110] Ignys I, Bartkowiak M, Baczyk I, Targonska B, Krawczynski M IV. Food allergy in pathogenesis of chronic abdominal pain in children. Pediatr Pol 1995;70(4):307-11.

[111] Pelto L, Salminen S, Lilius EM, Nuutila J, Isolauri E. Milk hypersensitivity-key to poorly defined gastrointestinal symptoms in adults. Allergy 1998;53(3):307-10.

[112] Read NW, Krejs GJ, Read MG, Santa Ana CA, Morawski SG, Fordtran JS. Chronic diarrhea of unknown origin. Gastroenterology 1980;78(2):264-71.

[113] Andersen AFR. Ulcerative colitis: an allergic phenomenon. Am J Dig Dis 1942;9:91-98.

[114] Rowe AH, Rowe A Jr. Chronic ulcerative colitis: atopic allergy in its etiology. Am J Gastroenterol 1960;34:49-60.

[115] Rider JA, Moeller HC. Food hypersensitivity in ulcerative colitis: further experience with an intramucosal test. Am J Gastroenterol 1962;37:497-507.

[116] Wright R, Truelove SC. A controlled therapeutic trial of various diets in ulcerative colitis. Br Med J 1965;2:138-141.

[117] Nowak-Wegrzyn A, Muraro A. Food protein-induced enterocolitis syndrome. Curr Opin Allergy Clin Immunol. 2009 Aug;9(4):371-7.

[118] Mindell EL, Hopkins V. Prescription Alternatives: Hundreds of safe, natural, prescription-free remedies to restore and maintain your health. Keats 1999.

[119] Seltzer S. Foods, and food and drug combinations, responsible for head and neck pain. Cephalalgia 1982 Jun;2(2):111-24.

[120] Staffieri D, Bentolila L, Leuit L. Hemiplegia and allergic symptoms following ingestion of certain foods. Ann Allergy 1951;10:38-39.

[121] Cooke RA. Allergic neuropathies. In: Cooke RA ed. Allergy in theory and practice. WB Saunders, 1947, 325-36.

[122] Breneman J. Basics of Food Allergy. Charles C Thomas 1978.

[123] Petitpierre M, Gumowski P, Girard JP. Irritable bowel syndrome and hypersensitivity to food. Ann Allergy 1985;54(6):538-40.

[124] Nanda R, James R, Smith H, et al. Food intolerance and the irritable bowel syndrome. Gut 1989;30:1099-1104.

[125] Antico A, Soana R, Clivio L, Baioni R. Irritable colon syndrome in intolerance to food additives. Minerva Dietol Gastroenterol 1989;35(4):219-24.

[126] Novembre E, Dini L, Bernardini R, Resti M, Vierucci A. Unusual reactions to food additives. Pediatr Med Chir 1992;14(1): 39-42.

[127] Golding DN. Is there an allergic synovitis? J R Soc Med 1990;83:312-4.

[128] Alexander P. It could be ALLERGY and it can be CURED. Ethicare Pty Ltd 1990.

[129] McKenna KE, Walsh MY, Burrows D. The Mekersson-Rosenthal syndrome and food additive hypersensitivity. Br J Dermatol 194;131:921-22.

[130] Randolph TG, Moss R W. An Alternative Approach to Allergies: The new field of clinical ecology unravels the environmental causes of mental and physical ills (revised edition). Perennial Library, Harper & Row 1990.

[131] Mandell M, Scanlon L W. Dr Mandell's 5-Day Allergy Relief System. Thomas Y Crowell 1979.

[132] Derebery MJ, Berliner KI.. Prevalence of allergy in Meniere's disease. Otolaryngol Head Neck Surg 2000;123(1Pt1):69-75.

[133] Derebery M J. Allergic management of Meniere's disease: an outcome study. Otolaryngol Head Neck Surg 2000;122(2):174-82.

[134] Haid CT, Watermeier D, Wolf SR, Berg M. Clinical survey of Meniere's disease: 574 cases. Acta Otolaryngol Suppl 1995;520 Pt 2:251-5.

[135] Balyeat RM, Brittain FL. Allergic migraine. Based on the study of fifty-five cases. Am J Med Sci 1930;180:212-221.

[136] Speer F. Allergy and migraine: a clinical study. Headache 1971;11:63-67.

[137] Grant EC. Food allergies and migraine. Lancet 1979;1(8123):966-9.

[138] Scheife RT, Hills JR. Migraine headache: signs and symptoms, biochemistry, and current therapy. Am J Hosp Pharm 1980;37:365-74.

[139] Merrett J, Peatfield RC, Rose FC, Merrett TG. Food related antibodies in headache patients. J Neurol Neurosurg Psychiatry 1983;46(8):738-42.

[140] Mansfield LE. Food allergy and headache. Whom to evaluate and how to treat. Postgrad Med 1988;83(7):46-51,55.

[141] Lucarelli S, Frediani T, Zingoni AM, Ferruzzi F, Giardini O, Quintieri F, Barbato M, D'Eufemia P, Cardi E. Food allergy and infantile autism. Panminerva Med 1995;37(3):137-41.

[142] Mylek D. Migraine as one of the symptoms of food allergy. Pol Tyg Lek 1992;20-27;47(3-4):89-91.

[143] Wantke F, Gotz M, Jarisch R. The histamine-free diet. Hautarzt 1993;44(8):512-6.

[144] Leira R, Rodriguez R. Diet and migraine. Rev Neurol 1996;24:534-8.

[145] Wray D. Gluten-sensitive recurrent aphthous stomatitis. Dig Dis Sci 1981;26:737-740.

[146] Hay KD, Reade PC. The use of an elimination diet in the treatment of recurrent aphthous ulceration of the oral cavity. Oral Surg 1984;57:504-507.

[147] Wright A, Ryan FP, Willingham SE, et al. Food allergy or intolerance in severe recurrent aphthous ulceration of the mouth. Br Med J 1986;292:1237-1238.

[148] Gerrard JW, Richardson JS, Donat J. Neuropharmacological evaluation of movement disorders that are adverse reactions to specific foods. Int J Neurosci 1994;76(1-2):61-9.

[149] Mandell M, Scanlon L W. Dr Mandell's 5-Day Allergy Relief System. Thomas Y Crowell 1979.

[150] Murray MT, Pizzorno JT. Encyclopaedia of Natural Medicine. Rocklin, CA: Prima Publishing; 1998.

[151] Kruger PG, Nyland HI. The role of mast cells and diet in the onset and maintenance of multiple sclerosis: a hypothesis. Med Hypothesis 1995;44(1):66-69.

[152] Sandberg DH, McIntosh RM, Bernstein CW, et al. Severe steroid-responsive nephrosis associated with hypersensitivity. Lancet 1977;1:388-391.

[153] Gaboardi F, Perletti L, Cambie M, Mihatsch MJ. Dermatitis herpetiformis and nephrotic syndrome. Clin Nephrol 1983, 20: 49-51.

[154] Lagrue G, Heslan JM, Belghiti D, Sainte-Laudy J, Laurent J. Basophil sensitization for food allergens in idiopathic nephrotic syndrome. Nephron 1986;42(2):123-7.

[155] Howanietz H, Lubec G. Idiopathic nephrotic syndrome, treated with steroids for five years, found to be allergic reaction to pork. Lancet 1985;2:450.

[156] Lagrue G, Laurent J, Rostoker G. Food allergy and idiopathic nephrotic syndrome. Kidney Int Suppl 1989;27:S147-51.

[157] Laurent J, Lagrue G. Dietary manipulation for idiopathic nephrotic syndrome. A new approach to therapy. Allergy 1989;44(8):599-603.

[158] Laurent J, Rostoker G, Robeva R, et al. Is adult idiopathic nephrotic syndrome food allergy? Value of oligoantigenic diets. Nephron 1987;47:7-11.

[159] Laurent J, Wierzbicki N, Rostoker G, Lang P, Lagrue G. Idiopathic nephrotic syndrome and food hypersensitivity. Value of an exclusion diet. Arch Fr Pediatr 1988;45(10):815-9.

[160] Bircher AJ, Van Melle G, Haller E, Curty B, Frei PC. IgE to food allergens are highly prevalent in patients allergic to pollens, with and without symptoms of food allergy. Clin Exp Allergy 1994;24:367-74.

[161] Amlot PL, Kemeny DM, Zachary C, Parks P, Lessof MH. Oral allergy syndrome (OAS): symptoms of IgE mediated hypersensitivity to foods. Clin Allergy 1987;17:33-8.

[162] Abraham G E . Nutritional factors in the etiology of the pre-menstrual tension syndrome. Journal Reprod Med 1983;28(7):446-64.

[163] Abraham G E. Management of the pre-menstrual tension syndromes: Rationale for a nutritional approach. In: Blond J (ed). 1986 A Year in Nutritional medicine. Keats 1986.

[164] Wurtman JJ, Brzezinski A, Wurtman RJ, Laferrere. Effect of nutrient intake on premenstrual depression. Am J Obst & Gyn 1989;161:1228-34

[165] Douglas JM. Psoriasis and diet. Calif Med 1980;133:5.

[166] Michaelsson G, Gerden B, Hagforsen E, Nilsson B, Pihl-Lundin I, Kraaz W, Hjelmquist G, Loof L. Psoriasis patients with antibodies to gliadin can be improved by a gluten-free diet. Br J Dermatol 2000;142(1):44-51.

[167] Nsouli TM, Nsouli SM, Linde RE, et al. Role of food allergy in serious otitis media. Ann Allergy 1994;73:215-219.

[168] Viscomi GJ. Allergic secretory otitis media: an approach to management. Laryngoscope 1975;85:751-758.

[169] Bernstein JM, Lee J, Conboy K, Ellis E, Li P. Further observations on the role of IgE-mediated hypersensitivity in recurrent otitis media with effusion. Otolaryngol Head Neck Surg 1985;93(5):611-5.

[170] Rousquet J, Chanez P, Michel F-B. The respiratory tract and food hypersensitivity. In: Metcalfe DD, Sampson HA, Simon RA. (eds) Food Allergy: Adverse reactions to foods and food additives, 2nd ed. Blackwell Science 1997.

[171] Lutz E G. Restless legs, anxiety and caffeinism. J Clin Psychiatry 1978; 693-8.

[172] Pelikan Z, Pelikan-Filipek M. Bronchial response to the food ingestion challenge. Ann Allergy 1987;58:164-172.

[173] Pastorello E et al. Evaluation of allergic etiology in perennial rhinitis. Ann Allergy 1985;55:854-56.

[174] Freedman BJ. Asthma induced by sulphur dioxide, benzoate and tartrazine contained in orange drinks. Clin Allergy 1977;7:407-415.

[175] Sampson H, Eigenmann PA. Allergic and non-allergic rhinitis: Food allergy and intolerance. In: Mygind N, Naclerio R, eds. Allergic and non-allergic rhinitis. Copenhagen: Munksgaard, 1997.

[176] Cingi C, Demirbas D, Songu M. Allergic rhinitis caused by food allergies. Eur Arch Otorhinolaryngol. 2010 Sep;267(9):1327-35.

[177] Kok YO, Yeoh KH, Wang DY. Effect of Diet Control in Food-Induced Allergic Rhinitis. Otolaryngol Head Neck Surg August 2010 vol. 143 no. 2 suppl P273-P274

[178] Raphael G, Raphael MH, Kaliner M. Gustatory rhinitis: a syndrome of food-induced rhinorrhea. J Allergy Clin Immunol 1989;83(1):110-5.

[179] Armanini D, Bonanni G, Palmero M. Reduction of serum testosterone in men by licorice. N Eng J Med 1999;341(15):1158.

[180] Spector S. The role of allergy in sinusitis in adults. J Allergy Clin Immunol. 1992;90:518-520.

[181] Nsouli TM, Nsouli SM, Linde RE, et al. Role of food allergy in serious otitis media. Ann Allergy 1994;73:215-219.

[182] Okudaira, H; Ito, K; Miyamoto, T et al. Evaluation of new system for the detection of IgE antibodies (ImmunoCAP®) in atopic disease. Arerugi; 1991;40(5):544-545.

[183] Kahn A, Mozin MJ, Rebuffat E et al. Milk intolerance in children with persistent sleeplessness: a prospective double blind crossover evaluation. Pediatrics 1989;84:595-603.

[184] Brien J A, Sigma. Ototoxicity associated with salicylates: A brief review. Drug Saf 1993;9(2):143-8.

[185] Cazals Y. Auditory sensori-neural alterations induced by salicylate. Prog Neurobiol 2000;(6):583-631.

[186] deBartolo H M Jr. Zinc and diet for tinnitus. Am Journal Otol 1989;10(3):256.

[187] Atherton DJ. Diagnosis and management of skin disorders caused by food allergy. Ann Allergy 1984;53(6Pt2):623-8.

[188] Swain A , Dutten SP, Truswell AS. Salicylates in Food. J Am Dietetic Assoc 1985;85(8).

[189] Juhlin L. Additives and chronic urticaria. Ann Allergy 1987;59:119-23.

[190] Henz BM, Zuberbier T. Most chronic urticaria is food-dependent, and not idiopathic. Exp Dermatol 1998;7(4):139-42.

[191] Zuberbier T, Chantraine-Hess S, Hartmann K, Czarnetzki BM. Pseudoallergen-free diet in the treatment of chronic urticaria. Acta Derm Venereol 1995 ;75(6):484-7. And Zuberbier T, Czarnetzki BM. High response rate to additive-free diet in chronic urticaria. Br J Dermatol 1996;134(6):1159.

[192] Verschave A, Stevens E, Degreef H. Pseudo-allergen-free diet in chronic urticaria. Dermatologica 1983;167(5):256-9.

[193] Rudzki E, Czubalski K, Grzywa Z. Detection of urticaria with food additives intolerance by means of diet. Dermatologica 1980;161:57-62.

[194] Montano Garcia ML, Orea M. Frequency of urticaria and angioedema induced by food additives. Rev Alerg Mex 1989;36(1):15-8.

[195] Veien NK, Krogdahl A. Cutaneous vasculitis induced by food additives. Acta Derm Venereol 1991;71(1):73-4.

[196] Businco L, Falconieri P, Bellioni-Businco B, Bahna SL. Severe food-induced vasculitis in two children. Pediatr Allergy Immunol. 2002 Feb;13(1):68-71.

[197] Dunn DW, Snyder CH. Benign paroxysmal vertigo of childhood. Am J Dis Child 1976;130:1099-100.

[198] Duke WW. Meniere's syndrome caused by allergy. JAMA 1923;34:645-47.

3 Food Intolerance and Food Allergy

Over the last few years more and more information on allergies has become available but information on food intolerance is still sparse—the subject is often covered as part of a discussion on allergy but leaves out vast amounts of information that you need to know. I suspect that part of the reason for this neglect of food intolerance is because of difficulties with definition.

In the late to mid 1920s a more rigid definition of allergy began to appear and although doctors may have found this more "scientific" it effectively drew boundaries that have led to food intolerance problems often being ignored and, at times, even denied. Older definitions along the lines of allergy "is an unwanted reaction in the body or mind caused by a food or chemical" quite clearly encompassed what we now know as food intolerance. So don't be fooled—the term "food intolerance" does not refer to a less serious problem.

I use the term "food intolerance" to refer to adverse reactions caused by a food, naturally occurring food chemical or food additive. You will also see the same type of reactions referred to as "food sensitivity" and "food hypersensitivity"—this is simply because there is no single accepted term for what are classed as non-allergic reactions to food.

The difference between food allergy and food intolerance is primarily one of evidence in the blood. It used to also be the case that anaphylactic reactions were thought to only take place if an allergy was present. Unfortunately that is not the case anymore and anaphylactic reactions have been experienced by individuals with an intolerance of food additives such as sulphites[1] and nitrates[2].

Soutter et al found that food intolerance is more likely to be a reaction to chemical substances found in many foods rather than the individual foods themselves. Symptoms are dose-related and may be cumulative from eating a range of foods containing the same substance. There can be a single symptom or a combination of a number of symptoms and these can vary over time. Reactions can take place within thirty minutes or up to forty eight hours after eating the problem food. They also found that preservatives and salicylates are the most likely to cause reactions but the range of substances that can affect a sensitive person varies from individual to individual.[3]

Other research has found that individuals react to various foods but when tested are not "allergic" so food intolerance, although often linked with food chemicals, can also be to any individual food. Future research may identify further chemicals that cause problems and clear this issue up but for the moment it is not known for definite what the actual cause is.

If your body cannot tolerate a particular food, or one of its ingredients, then you will experience an unwanted reaction. The type of symptoms that arise are very individual specific and it is not possible to say that, for example, apples will cause headaches or milk will cause stomach problems. They may do, but they may also cause other symptoms. The simple truth is that any reaction can be provoked by any food.

It is also important to understand that food intolerance is not the same as food allergy. In the case of an allergic reaction there is an immunological response that can be measured and "seen" in the blood. No such method of testing exists for food intolerance.

The safest, and most accurate, way of detecting food intolerance is by using an elimination diet that first removes the suspect food, in all its forms, from your diet and is then reintroduced. If there is a negative reaction, that food, for whatever reason, is not safe for you to eat. If, after a period of time, there is no reaction then the food is safe, for you, to eat. Without the aid of an appropriate blood test it is unlikely that you will know if your reaction can be defined as an allergy or intolerance problem. The situation is further complicated by the fact that reactions caused by allergy and intolerance are very similar.

In some instances it is possible to identify the cause of the intolerance. For example, many people cannot tolerate milk because they are lacking in the enzyme lactase which is essential for the digestion of lactose, the sugar found in milk. We also know that some substances, such as caffeine, act like drugs and we can point to a problem of overuse or overdose. Sadly, for most other forms of intolerance the situation is not as clear cut and if you find yourself intolerant of a food the odds are seriously stacked against you knowing the reason for your intolerance. Vatn suggests that the mechanism behind food intolerance is one of the greatest enigmas of modern medicine.[4]

Although this may be cause for concern for doctors and researchers, it need not concern you. Maybe one day they will ascertain the reasons, and maybe even find solutions, but until then you can still get healthier by avoiding the food or foods that cause you a problem. It is after all the case that many drugs have proved effective at removing or relieving symptoms yet little is actually known as to how some of these work—

this is especially the case with drugs used to treat so called mental illnesses.

Testing Methods

An allergic reaction leads to an immunological response that can be measured and "seen" in the blood. No such method of identification, and hence testing, exists for food intolerance. The safest and most accurate, way of detecting food intolerance is by using an elimination diet that first removes the food, in all its forms, from your diet and is then reintroduced.

The three main types of medically approved allergy testing are:

- The Skin Prick Test where the suspected allergen is injected just under the surface of the skin and the reaction is observed. Not all allergies can be identified by this method.

- Patch Testing where the test substance is applied to the skin, covered with a patch and left in place for a period of time (up to 48 hours). Mainly used to establish if there is a contact allergy leading to some form of skin rash.

- Blood testing to detect the presence of an antibody called IgE in the blood. IgE is the substance that causes allergic reactions. Different substances produce specific IgEs and this enables the test to identify more than one allergen. Results are expressed on a grade that indicates how much IgE specific to the substance you tested for, is present in your blood. The higher the grade the more likely you are to be allergic.

The blood test used to only be available through the medical profession but there are some organisations that will now carry out these tests for you. You should note that a negative test does not 100% rule out an allergy. It is, also, possible to have a positive IgE test when you have either outgrown the allergy or not yet developed any symptoms. IgE testing will not identify a food intolerance problem.

The other main method of testing is a "food challenge" (sometimes called "oral challenge"). During a food challenge test, you are given the test food usually in gradually increasing amounts to see how you react. Whilst this is one of the most effective methods of testing for an adverse reaction to a food the medical profession does not generally like it as only one food can be tested at each appointment. It is also problematic for some doctors as they will not be able to say if the reaction is an allergic one or an intolerance one and for some medics the "correct" label is of great importance.

Other tests are available and some of these claim to identify food intolerances as well as allergies. The ALCAT test measures platelet aggregation and changes in white blood cells after mixing whole blood with various food extracts. Hoj[5] found it to be fairly reliable for identifying reactions to food additives but Fell et al found it far less successful in the testing of food allergies.[6]

Provocative testing, using dilutions of food extracts are used by some practitioners and a similar procedure is used to "neutralise" or desensitise allergies. Although the efficacy of food extract injection therapy has been demonstrated in a double-blind study by Miller[7] others including Lehman[8] failed to find a beneficial effect.

What you need to know before parting with your money is that food intolerance does not cause a specific response in the body that can be measured. Yes, it does sometimes cause a fluctuation in the pulse that can be detected and sometimes a measurable IgG but not always. Also, no one substance is produced in the blood that can be used to measure all forms of food intolerance. Given that *any* food can cause *any* reaction and that your food problems could in fact be being caused by food chemicals these tests need to approached with some degree of caution.

A common food allergy test, in commercial use, measures IgG in the blood. Kleine-Tebbe et al note that, whilst many of the samples showed positive IgG4 results, there were no corresponding clinical symptoms. This, combined with the lack of convincing evidence for histamine-releasing properties of IgG4 in humans, and the lack of any controlled studies on the diagnostic value of IgG4 testing in food allergy, call into question the value of these type of tests.

They argue that food-specific IgG4 does not indicate (imminent) food allergy or food intolerance. What it does indicate is a physiological response of the immune system to food components. They conclude that these type of tests should not be used to identify food related problems. It would seem that presence of IgG4 may only indicate that you have recently eaten the food identified and that your body has reacted as expected.[9]

One of my concerns with these tests is that some people come away with a very long list of foods to be avoided. If they avoided all of these foods their diets would be very restricted. My own view is that, if this type of test is used as a diagnostic tool, it still needs to be followed up by individual testing of the identified foods (by eliminating the food and then reintroducing it) to confirm whether they are in fact causing a problem.

An excellent study by Joneja identifies the difficulties in testing for food allergy and especially for food intolerance. She concludes that no single method of testing can identify all problem foods or the constituents within the food because the immunological, physiological and biochemical reactions that effect food sensitivity are so diverse. Elimination and challenge testing often provide the most accurate results.[10]

Allergy testing is often seen as being well proven, scientific and accurate. In contrast, food intolerance testing is seen as unscientific and unproven. But just how accurate is allergy testing? Well, that depends... For example, skin prick tests are performed to identify the causes of allergy but when compared to results from oral challenges there has always been a great degree of inconsistency. Doctors have never been able to explain why this should be the case.

A study of skin prick testing by Kim et al goes a long way to providing some answers. Quite simply, the results from skin prick tests significantly improves when fresh food is used for the test rather than commercial allergen extracts. The study focused on patients with atopic dermatitis and the allergens investigated were milk, egg white, egg yolk, and soya bean. What they found was that when you compare fresh food samples and commercial allergens they are different in structure. Most significantly some of the protein elements implicated in allergic reactions are missing in the commercial samples.[11]

Before you rush of to your allergist and demand a different type of skin prick test it is worth noting that even though the fresh foods resulted in a greater degree of accuracy the percentages still did not reach the seventies. It would appear that oral food challenges and use of elimination diets are more accurate methods of testing.

Similar findings have emerged from other studies. Vojdani argues that one of the reasons traditional food sensitivity testing fails is that it does not reflect a real world non-raw food diet. The problem is not only that a food can change when processed but that the effect it has in the body can also be different when it is combined with other foods. So, a person "who is allergic to ketchup may not have an immune reaction to raw tomato". Normal testing methods would not identify or resolve that individual's problems.[12]

The reality is that identifying food related problems can be difficult. In some instances, the food culprit is very clear, in others a lot of work has to be done to find the problem makers. In yet other cases, the problem ingredient can be so hidden that it can easily be overlooked and missed. A case described by Leduc et al illustrates this—it was thought that an individual was allergic to wheat in sausages and pork pies but allergy testing to wheat was negative. It was only when the actual real-time ingredient, in this case wheat isolate, was tested that a positive reaction was confirmed.[13]

If you have ever suspected that you have an allergy and been sent for tests that have all turned out negative and been told there is nothing wrong with you, when you know there is, then don't despair—you are probably food intolerant.

Just because you can't measure it doesn't mean it doesn't exist.

In 1991 Sloper et al presented their findings on the links
 between eczema and food in children and reported on their immunological findings. Although they were able to observe that eczema, for many of the children, improved significantly during the diet and became worse on food challenges, the clinical outcome of food elimination could not be predicted by the initial skin prick test results, serum immunoglobulins, total or food-specific IgE, or complex IgG or IgE. This study

sends a very clear message that allergy tests are not, always, enough.[14]

What you have to understand is that an allergic reaction can be caused by a very small amount of the problem food, in respect of intolerance this is not generally the case. Food chemicals, such as salicylate and solanine, build up in the body and it is only when the individual's tolerance is breached that problems appear. Challenge testing with a concentrated form of the chemical can be misleading as most are cumulative in the body and the amount varies from day to day. A positive reaction is of no help in ascertaining the level you can in fact tolerate.

We all want a quick and easy answer but the reality is that this is not always possible. If you do use one of these tests and are presented with a list of foods to avoid, do not accept the list as definitive proof of your problems. By far the wisest course of action would be then to test each of these foods using an elimination diet. If you don't do this you could be restricting your diet far too severally and unnecessarily.

Why bother with an elimination diet when you know someone who has had massive improvements by following the advice given as a result of one of these tests? Because your health matters and what works for one person will not necessarily work for someone else. Two of the most common foods that people are asked to eliminate are milk and wheat and I think you will be a rare individual not to experience some positive health changes if you eliminate these but this is not always indicative of a food intolerance problem. Wheat and milk are two foods that are consumed daily, often at each meal, and removing them from the diet often leads to some improvement. It is possible that your body is simply enjoying a rest, that you are intolerant of gluten or are lactose deficient or that you have a problem with amines and so on.

In 2008 undercover researchers for *Which?* trialled various tests that claim to diagnose food intolerances through analysis of blood samples or strands of hair, changes in electric current, or resistance to pressure applied to their legs or arms (the tests cost between £45 and £275 each). The researchers had one medically confirmed allergy and one food intolerance between them yet the tests diagnosed one hundred and eighty three intolerances. They also found that identical blood and hair samples sent under different names to the same company produced different test results. Their advice to people who are concerned that they may have an allergy or intolerance was "to keep a record of symptoms and a food diary, and speak to their GP".[15]

Soutter et al in their study of food allergy and food intolerance in children state that food chemical intolerance can only be assessed by means of an appropriate elimination diet and challenge protocol. Blood and skin tests are not helpful or appropriate.[16] Sadly few doctors, allergists or other health practitioners are aware of the problems these chemicals can cause.

Elimination diets are the only accurate way of determining most forms of food intolerance and a simple easy to use system is outlined below in the *Seven Step Plan*.

Before you even think about following the plan you should consult with your doctor and ensure that there is no underlying illness.

The Seven Step Plan

The Seven Step Plan is a simple and easy to use system for identifying food intolerance problems. It is designed to help you take things at your own pace and to place as little stress on your body as possible.

Step 1: Decide to take some action

In many ways this step is the hardest. Change is something that is constantly happening within and around us yet our naturally tendency is to resist change. This is a normal human response but one we need to be aware of when reviewing our diet and health.

In respect of health, we are more used to being told what to do rather than choosing a course of action for ourselves. If a doctor says there is nothing wrong with us, then, despite our symptoms, we accept the diagnosis and often interpret it as meaning that there is nothing that can be done. As you are reading this book and have reached this stage. You are probably fed up with being ill, overweight or depressed and you will probably have already tried many other avenues of help. Please don't despair—I managed to find a route to better health after more than thirty six years of being ill and miserable. If I can do it then I have every faith that others can also do it.

I am, however, not offering a quick fix—I wish I could—rather a slow evaluation of your situation and a move towards finding the diet that works for you which, when found, will change your life.

What you most need to know and remember is that the only true expert on you is yourself. Your instincts may have become a little clouded but they are still there and will re-emerge to help you. I used to laugh when I read advice like "listen to your stomach" or liver or some other organ—I couldn't differentiate one from another. I also could not trust my inner voice about whether a food was good for me or not—it was all simply food, in the shops and therefore safe. It was not something I thought about except in terms of whether it was "healthy".

The self-preservation instinct does re-emerge when you start to remove the layers of toxins and you do come to be able to listen to what your body is saying, whether it is because it needs something different or needs you to stop eating something. This will happen for you but for now trust more in observation and logic than feelings.

However, we are not going to completely ignore feelings. Before you decide to take some action you need to be clear about what it is you are trying to change. Your overall goal will be to find the ideal healthy diet for you but the other details will be very specific to you. Start by writing out how you feel about your health and how you feel about what you have read so far in this book.

This will be useful for you to later look back on—as you get better you will begin to forget how awful things were and having something in writing will boost your confidence and help you keep going. If you don't know where to start then take a pen and some paper, sit somewhere quiet, take a few slow deep breaths, and simply begin to write. Don't worry if you start writing gibberish. Just let the words flow—this is for your eyes only.

Why bother? Not feeling well, whether physically or mentally, takes a massive toll on us especially if we simply have to get on with all the usual demands of life—work, family, housework, social commitments etc... You will have strong feelings about your health and it is better to get these out than to keep them locked inside. You may be surprised at what you discover.

Later... Take some more paper and list all your symptoms. For each symptom note any diagnosis and treatment and how effective it has been. Identify the symptoms that just do not seem to change no matter what you do (and this can include changes you have made in your diet). Now decide that you want to take some action. Write a note to yourself promising yourself that you are going to do the best you can to make yourself better by changing your diet.

Step 2: Simplify your diet

Food, even in its simplest form, is a complex substance. Combine a whole range of foods and additives together and you increase the complexity.

If you are sensitive to any foods or food chemicals you need to find out which ones. To find out you will have to test foods. In order to test foods you will need to eat them in their simplest, most natural form possible. The more complex your diet the harder it will be to unravel a food intolerance problem. It is essential that you simplify your diet.

Reactions to products such as chocolate, a chicken salad sandwich, steak pie, oven ready chips (fries), or lentil burgers tell us nothing. We need to know which ingredient in these products brought about the reaction. If we don't then it is likely that our problems will recur. To clarify let us look at a couple of examples.

A reaction to milk chocolate could be a reaction to milk, cocoa, cocoa butter, vegetable fat, a flavouring (usually some form of vanilla —natural or manmade), the type of sweetener used, or soya (in the form of lecithin).

A reaction to a shop bought chicken salad sandwich will leave you unsure as to whether the problem was one of the ingredients in the bread that was used, the chicken, one of the salad ingredients, one of the ingredients in the margarine, or one of the ingredients in the salad dressing.

You need to simplify your diet. If, for example, you had made the chicken salad sandwich at home you would have known exactly what went it and you could have left out the dressing so that the sandwich contained fewer ingredients.

The complexity of ready-made food is astounding. If I make shepherd's pie at home it will contain minced beef, onions, possibly some herbs, potato and oil. Yet if I buy a ready-made one it will also contain a mix of food additives that are there to ensure the food maintains its structure, texture and taste. It may also contain a stock that has many ingredients and thickening agents. Suddenly my body is faced with having to digest and deal with thirty plus chemicals rather than just a few.

If you don't simplify your diet you will find it very difficult to identify problem foods, will find yourself getting very confused and eliminating foods that are okay for you whilst eating others that are not. This is a very common problem. Save yourself time and misery by truly simplifying your diet before testing for food intolerance problems.

By far the easiest way to simplify your diet is to reduce the amount of processed food you eat and to eliminate, as much as you can, food additives. Your goal should be to eat your usual diet in as natural a form as possible. Ideally you would remove all processed food and all additives but we live in a busy world and even with the best of intentions you will find this difficult but aim to get as near to it as you can—don't sell yourself short.

We have become very dependent on processed food and at first it is daunting to consider breaking this dependency. Make the change gradually. Do not make any drastic change to your diet—simply try replace the more complex foods with similar ones with fewer ingredients. There are lots of ways in which you can do this. For example:

- Plain crisps often contain only potatoes, vegetable oil and salt. Flavoured crisps are far more complex as they include a variety of flavourings and colours.

- Breakfast cereals can contain colours and preservatives. Choose a similar one that contains fewer ingredients or make your own muesli from ingredients purchased at a health food shop.

- Cereal bars are often seen as a healthy option but many contain artificial flavours rather than real fruit, sugar and can be high in fat. Choose bars that only contain cereals and fruit.

- Chocolates can be packed with added flavourings, colours, emulsifiers, raising agents, biscuit pieces and other ingredients. Choose ones that have the fewest number of ingredients. A simple chocolate bar will have far fewer ingredients than one that has been flavoured or had other things added.

- Sweets (candies) can be extremely complex products but there are now some on the market that contain very few, or no, artificial colours and flavours. The brighter, more unnatural the colour the greater the number of additives.

- Fizzy drinks can often be a cocktail of chemicals—check the labels and choose the one with the least or, if you feel ready, change to drinking mineral water or try adding a small amount of fresh fruit juice, such as orange or lemon, to some sparkling mineral water). Try avoid all artificial sweeteners.

- Nuts can be bought in their original form without added oils, salts and flavourings.

A few tips:

- Go as natural as you can.

- Cook your own meat and do not buy processed meats like salamis and sausages. If you absolutely have to eat these products search out the ones with the fewest ingredients.

- If you eat yoghurt then buy the natural variety and add your own fruit.

- Avoid tinned vegetables and fruit—stick with fresh or use frozen.

- Never buy ready-made meals as these are incredibly complex. Buy the ingredients instead and make your own (if you're not a cook then buy a cook book and you'll soon be on a journey of discovery to the true taste of food).

- Dishes requiring sauces are easy enough to make if you take the time to find out how. A tomato based sauce using tomatoes, onion, garlic and a sprinkling of herbs takes only minutes longer to prepare than a shop bought one.

- If you eat sandwiches for lunch then make your own rather than taking your chance at the sandwich bar or eating too much in a cafe or restaurant. If you are interested in losing weight this will also help you reduce your calories without trying—most of us do not use the amounts of margarine and dressings that a commercial outlet does.

- Margarines can be highly coloured—choose the one with the smallest number of ingredients and preferably one that tells you which type of oils are actually used. The term "vegetable oil" can mean one or a combination of many different types.

- If you have a freezer, cook meals ahead and freeze them.

- If you have to eat away from home choose the simplest menu option and avoid sauces.

- Always have a low additive snack food or fruit with you.

- Avoid buying food on impulse.

The easiest way of helping yourself is to plan ahead. Sit down and work out the meals you will eat for the week and buy accordingly. If you leave the decision until half an hour before you need to make a meal your options will be limited and you are more likely to succumb to heavily processed food.

Takes too much time? It doesn't really. If you don't plan and prepare you probably spend more time each day waiting for your food to be cooked at take-outs or rushing around supermarkets trying to decided what to have.

Still seems difficult? Don't worry and don't panic. I am not expecting you to make a total change overnight. Gradually decrease the amount of processed food in your diet. Do not, however, change the basic structure of your diet. Eat the same type of foods you were eating only in a more natural and simpler form. So if you are vegetarian do not suddenly start eating meat. If you have never eaten nuts then do not start. If you have always avoided lettuce do not start eating it. And so on.

Food additives

I am frequently asked why I am so keen that you reduce the number of additives as surely these are safe. Well, yes some maybe but some may not be. Each country has regulatory bodies that deal with the safety and regulation of how additives are used in food. The quotes below from the UK government are a typical official view.

Additives allowed in the UK are "considered safe for almost everyone... There are a few additives to which a few people may react badly. But this is not good enough reason to ban such additives: substances in everyday food like milk, wheat, oranges or strawberries upset far more people. The value of the additive to everyone is weighed against the upset it may cause to a small number of people".[17]

So safe for some but not safe for all. The truth is that you can be intolerant of any additive or group of similar additives. As it is rarely possible to test these in isolation from food it is far better to begin your food intolerance testing with real food. As Hannuksela and Haahtela point out, food additives seldom provoke true allergic (i.e. measurable) reactions. Intolerance is more likely to take place and this type of individual intolerance may change and fluctuate from time to time.[18]

Additives have been implicated in a wide range of health problems including behaviour problems, bloating, headaches, gastrointestinal problems, respiratory difficulties, and skin problems. Antico and Di Berardino found additives to be a frequent cause of skin complaints.[19] Leira and Rodriguez found them implicated in migraines.[20] Novembre et al saw them induce symptoms in other organs including the joints and central nervous system, symptoms included over activity, concentration and learning difficulties, and depression.[21] Rowe and Rowe found they caused hyperactivity in some children.[22] Kanny et al demonstrated a link between additives and dermatitis.[23]

Even the additives that are classed as "natural" have been implicated in health problems. For example, Ebo et al describe the case of a fifty-eight year old man who experienced four episodes, in three years, of severe anaphylaxis with urticaria, angioedema and finally loss of consciousness within a few minutes after eating a sandwich or toast with Gouda cheese. Testing confirmed that the problem was annatto (E160b).[24]

Scurlock et al outline the case of a young girl who experienced anaphylaxis after eating gummy bears. She was tested for allergy to the various ingredients but all results were negative. The authors concluded that she was reacting to the added "natural and artificial flavors" but because the manufacturers would not disclose the ingredients within these it was not possible for them to identify the exact culprit. The authors write: "Currently, vendors are reluctant to reveal the variable components of these flavorings. In light of the potentially life-threatening complications that can ensue from consumption of these products, cooperation with industry and improved labelling of all ingredients is essential".[25]

The list goes on and on... Food additives can cause serious problems for some people. They also make your diet incredibly complex and that is why I want you to reduce them. Basically if it was not something you would place in your food when cooking at home then avoid it. Not only will you simplify your diet but you will also discover how food is supposed to taste. You need to be aware that many additives are present in food but are not listed amongst the ingredients (this may vary from country to country).

Some of the ways in which additives are hidden in food as well as other labelling problems are listed below:

- Some food ingredients need only be identified by a generic term (such as oil or spices) and additives used in such ingredients need not be named.

- Additives contained in ingredients of a food rarely need to listed unless they perform a technological function in the final foodstuff.

- Flavourings do not have to be individually listed only the term "flavouring" need appear. There are more than 3000 flavourings in use. You will have no idea which one has been used, what it is made from or how it was produced.

- Terms such as "vegetable oil" and "sugar" can be potentially misleading. "Sugar" could be cane, beet or corn sugar and could change over time as the manufacturer decides which is the best option for him to use (usually the cheapest). Vegetable oil could be rapeseed, corn, soya, sunflower and so on–it is probably best to use an oil that is just, for example, sunflower or olive oil.

- Modified starch frequently appears on labels but we have no knowledge of the source and this could again vary from batch to batch depending on economic factors at the time of manufacture.

- Additives are manufactured substances but their identifying name and number provide us with no indication as to the origin of the substance. This can cause problems for some individuals. For example: Anyone sensitive to aspirin is best avoiding azo dyes which are often used in the production of food colourings. Someone with a lactose intolerance may need to avoid, among others, E325 which is the sodium salt of lactic acid.

- Some food and drinks are exempt from listing their ingredients including: alcoholic drinks and some, including beer, lager, cider and wine, can contain a number of additives; bakery items such as bread, cakes, pastries and cookies; take-away and fast foods. Consume any of these foods and you will not know what you are eating.

- Additives used as processing aids need not be listed. These include powders and greases to stop foods sticking, anti-caking agents to stop powders forming lumps, acids that produce raising agents, and bleaches. In theory only a residue will remain in the food you bought but you will not know what has been used or how much of it has been left behind in the product you're eating.

- The term "allergen free" is misleading as it only means that the food does not contain the substances on the current list of excluded allergens. The current EU list is: gluten containing grains, crustaceans, eggs, fish, peanuts, soybeans, milk, most nuts, celery, mustard, sesame seeds, lupin, molluscs, and sulphur dioxide and sulphites at certain concentrations.

The complexity of any processed food is further increased by hidden additives—the sausages with fifteen listed ingredients could in reality contain more than thirty different substances. If you bought some mince and rolled it into sausage shapes you would be providing your body with a less complex product to digest with just two ingredients—the meat and the oil you fry the "sausages" in.

The comfort of added vitamins could also, rather than helping, be hurting. BHT and BHA are frequently found in margarines and other vitamin-fortified foods. Feingold identified vitamins A, D and E as frequently containing BHT, one of the substances he identified as being linked with hyperactivity.[26]

It is also the case that for many additives there is a safe daily intake level known as the "Accepted Daily Intake" or ADI for short. Even if you knew the amounts you would not be able to gauge the amount you were ingesting as the amount per serving is not declared on labels and many substances do not have to declare the amounts available. For example, sulphites (E numbers 220 to 228) are frequently used in wines, beers and ciders—drink too much and you could exceed the ADI.[27,28] Likewise with antioxidants such as BHA, BHT, TBHQ and gallates—these are all commonly used in foods that contain fat, such as crisps and chips, and they do have ADIs.

Certainly as an individual, you would not be able to calculate the amount of BHA, for example, that you had ingested. Even if the exact amount was stated on each item and you did the calculation according to your weight and the other foods you had eaten that day that contained BHA you would still not have a complete picture. How much had you taken in from ingredients that had not been listed? Was there any on the packaging and if so what amount was likely to have migrated into the food you ate? Had any been used as a processing aid?

The scientist would say that you don't need this information as the amounts are negligible. But the reality is that these amounts can cause problems especially if they ingested daily on a long term basis and when you are trying to identify a food intolerance problem having these type of additives in your diet can seriously cloud the results for you.

Do you really want to be eating cocktails of chemicals whose effects we know so little about? If your answer is "no, but it is easier, convenient and probably okay", I know exactly how you feel.

Make the changes that you can but be aware of the potential problems. I will, later in this book, explain how to use a food diary that may help you pick up on some of these hidden problems.

As you make the changes you may begin to experience some improvements. If you do please make a note of them as the information could prove valuable later. And remember, even if you start to feel much better, this is only the beginning, better things are yet to come. If, however, you find yourself becoming more irritable, tired and feeling stressed stop and think before you revert back to your normal diet. Your body could just be detoxifying and this can take time.

Additives are thought to accumulate in the body so it can take some time for the body to eliminate them.[29] If you have had a problem with some food additives then your body could be experiencing withdrawal and this, not the change in your diet, could be making you feel ill. Persevere but please remember to eat the more natural versions of what you were eating rather than introducing foods unfamiliar to your body.

You need to stay at this stage for at least two weeks but you can stay here for as long as you like or need. If the improvements have been startling you may decide not to continue with the following stages, you can always do so later. If you have felt ill then you need to give yourself time to build up your strength and allow your body to continue with its elimination of built up toxins and healing before continuing with specific food tests. If there has been little or no change then press on to the next stage.

Step 3: Know what you are eating

Food intolerance is difficult to diagnose and, at the moment, the only accurate way is to eliminate foods from your diet and then reintroduce them. If you are doing this for more than one food or for any food chemical you will get confused. Don't assume you will be able to remember what you've eaten or how you felt—you won't.

Keep a food diary and keep it diligently. Not only will it help you keep track of the food you've eaten and how you felt but it will also help you monitor changes. I recently found one of my very early food diaries and was quite shocked at how ill I had been and also how complex my diet used to be. I had forgotten and it was a very helpful reminder especially as I was going through a bad reaction at the time.

Many people discover that they are food intolerant without the help of a doctor and when they present this information to the doctor they are not believed. This is understandable. If you have never witnessed for yourself a food reaction then you will be sceptical. One way of helping present the evidence to your doctor is by use of a food diary—he may still be sceptical but at least you have it down on paper and are not just waxing lyrical about the changes that have taken place. If you are going to use your food diary as evidence for your doctor do endeavour to keep it as clear and concise as possible. The more professional it looks the more he is going to be inclined to read it and, hopefully, accept your findings.

You can download a free print for yourself Food Diary from the Food Can Make You Ill Web site: www.foodcanmakeyouill.co.uk. You can also make your own—buy a notebook or paper and a binder. You will need one page for each day. Divide the day into three segments. Draw a line down the centre of the page, dividing it in two. List the food you eat on the left side and your symptoms on the right hand side. See the example page below.

As you need to list all the ingredients in every meal, you will find it easier if, at the back of your notebook, you keep a list of any complex foods that you eat and their ingredients. For example, if you eat muesli then in your complex foods list add "muesli" and list the ingredients fully—oats, wheat flakes, coconut, sunflower seeds, almonds, sultanas, hazelnuts and so on. Then when you eat muesli you only need to write "MUESLI".

Why so detailed? It can be extremely difficult to identify some food intolerance problems and a very detailed food diary can provide you with the clues that you need. By the way, a complex food is any one that contains more than one ingredient such as muesli, soup, biscuits, sauces, pastries. You should also note the brand name of the product. The example page lists all the complex foods in block capitals.

Day and Date: Saturday 6 July   **EXAMPLE**

	Morning
	Bad night's sleep. Uncomfortable all over – suspect restaurant meal last night.
Black Coffee (brand name)	
MUESLI with milk	
Coffee x 2 (with milk)	
Banana	Indigestion

	Afternoon
Jacket Potato with butter and cottage cheese (plain) Salad – tomato, cucumber, iceberg lettuce, cress, spring onion.	Felt better after lunch but energy dropped by 4 pm and I developed a terrible headache.
HEADACHE PILLS (brand name)	
Coffee x 2 (black)	
FLAPJACK (homemade)	

	Evening
Lamb chop grilled Brown rice (organic) – steamed, long grain. Stir fry veg – cabbage greens, mushrooms, bamboo shoots fried in cold pressed sunflower oil. VITAMIN E Coffee x 3 CHOCOLATE (brand name)	Mood quite low. Physically very tired but not sleepy.

Use your diary fully. List all ingredients of every meal and their scores (when applicable). Make a note of any medication you may be taking. Write down any changes whether positive or negative—include all physical and mental changes. If you get a cold, flu or tummy upset write it down so that you can try separate it from any other changes. Write down anything you feel is significant. For example, if you had a headache after being stuck in traffic for two hours note down that the journey was the probable cause.

Write up your diary every day. If you forget or find yourself too ill to do it then don't punish yourself or give up on the idea. Simply write down what you can remember and also why you didn't write it at the time—this could be vital information as many mental symptoms can be produced by food intolerance, most classically brain fogging and confusion.

Step 4: Develop a strategy

At this stage you need to decide on which you foods or food chemicals you are going to test. If you already have suspicions about certain foods then start with those. Check back over your food diary and see if any type of pattern is emerging—do remember that problems with food can manifest many hours, even days, after being eaten.

If you are still uncertain read through the sections on food chemicals and food problems. It is likely that at least one of these will leap out at you. If it doesn't think about the foods that you eat and have eaten in the past. Are there any you feel you just cannot live without? Unfortunately, this probably indicates a food addiction whose underlying cause is usually an intolerance problem. Remember any food can cause problems.

You may have refused certain types of food as a child but been made to eat them because they were "good for you" (children who are "picky" eaters could be signalling a food intolerance problem). You may know that some foods give you stomach problems or a hangover effect but because you enjoy them or they are "good for you" you keep on eating them.

Make a list of the foods or food chemicals you want to test and prioritise them—put the one you think is the most likely culprit at the top of your list and the reason why. Do not be tempted to try to eliminate more than one food or food chemical at a time. Rather than speeding up the process this will lead to confusion and cause additional stress to the body. Please, also, do not be tempted to fast and then introduce one food at a time. This places enormous stress on the body, leads to confusing results and the slow process of reintroducing foods can lead to a diet that does not sustain health. There is a time and place for fasting and this isn't it.

I receive many requests from people asking me where they should start and it is impossible for me to direct them, or you, to the specific food, foods or food chemicals that may be causing them or you a problem. You are a unique individual and what causes you a problem may be totally okay for someone else. As I've said before although a food may cause a certain type of reaction in some people it will not always cause this symptom.

However, I do understand how difficult starting out on this journey can be and I accept that you may need some further guidelines so, if you are truly uncertain as to where to begin, use the check list below to guide you. Find your main symptom and then read the corresponding sections in the book and see if any "speak" to you.

Acid reflux: caffeine, capsaicin.

Anxiety: caffeine, MSG, salicylate.

Asthma and breathing difficulties: benzoates, histamine, lectins, milk, MSG, sulphur and sulphites.

Behaviour problems: gluten, milk, salicylates, wheat.

Catarrh and sinus problems: milk, salicylates.

Depression: caffeine, gluten, grains, salicylate, sugar, wheat.

Fatigue: caffeine, MSG, wheat.

Gastrointestinal problems: amines, capsaicin, gluten, grains, lectins, legumes, milk, oxalic acid, purines, sulphur and sulphites, wheat.

Gout: purines.

High blood pressure: tyramine.

Hyperactivity: caffeine, salicylate.

Joint pain: gluten, lectins, purines, serotonin, solanine, wheat.

Kidney/bladder stones: oxalic acid, purines.

Migraines: amines, caffeine, histamine, phenylethylamine, serotonin, sugar and sweeteners, tannins, tyramine.

Mood swings: gluten, MSG, salicylate, solanine, sugar, tyramine, wheat.

Mouth problems: capsaicin, fruit, histamine.

Panic attacks: caffeine.

Restless legs: caffeine, grains, salicylate.

Skin problems: benzoates, fish, fruit, grains, histamine, milk, peanuts, salicylate, wheat.

Sleeping problems: caffeine, gluten, milk, salicylate.

Tics: caffeine, salicylate.

Tinnitus: salicylate, sugar and sweeteners.

If you still remain uncertain as to where to start then consider testing wheat and/or milk. I only suggest these as they are two foods that are often consumed many times a day. A "holiday" from either of them will not do you any harm. If there is any other food that you have eaten each and every day of your life then that food could also go on your suspect list. Dr Mumby identifies three main allergens for adults: wheat, dairy produce, and instant coffee. He writes: "If one were simply able to persuade the entire population to give up just these three foods, the change in the health of the nation would be dramatic".[30]

Be gentle, take it slowly.

At this stage you need to consult your doctor. Dr Michael Tettenborn a consultant paediatrician at the Frimley Children's Centre in Surrey, suggests that many doctors have been turned against dietary management because some people have made excessive claims about its potential impact and that their scepticism is fuelled by the range of tests in use by non-medical practitioners.[31] Bearing this in mind I have outlined a strategy that you can use in preparing for your appointment:

1. Make a list of the symptoms that concern you with details of how long these have been a problem.

2. List any treatments you have tried and their outcomes.

3. Make a few notes for yourself as to why you want to test for food intolerance—this will help give you confidence

when talking to your doctor (we all get nervous and if you are unwell your self confidence will be low).

4. Take the food diary you will be using—this will show your doctor how he can follow your progress. The food diary is going to be your way of presenting evidence.

5. If you want to take additional information along with you make sure it is information that is acceptable to your doctor. Many doctors are suspicious of information obtained on the Internet so ensure that you know the source of what you are presenting. Details of articles in medical journals are going to carry more weight than somebody's home page.

6. Remember that your doctor is an individual who has been trained in medicine—he is there to help not hinder you. If you are not happy with your doctor you always have the option of changing to another one.

7. Remember it is okay to ask questions, make suggestions and take notes.

8. If your doctor is obviously pushed for time then suggest you make an appointment for a longer session later.

9. Remember your doctor is a human being like you. He, like you and I, is not perfect. Your doctor does not know everything but then neither do you or I. Respect and co-operation are better than hostility and antagonism.

As unravelling illness can be a complex process I advocate the path of co-operation with the medical profession but I am also very aware that you may meet resistance. If at all possible seek help from another doctor or an alternative practitioner. If you do decide to go ahead with testing on your own please take extreme care when testing foods—it is always best to have someone else, who understands what you are doing, present just in case you have a severe problem. NEVER stop medication without your doctor's consent.

Once you have decided on your strategy then decide when you are going to begin the next step—eliminating the suspect foods. You can repeat the next three steps as many times as you need and at your own pace, returning to step two whenever you need.

Step 5: Eliminate suspect foods

The key to successfully eliminating a suspect food lies in planning. Know when you are going to start and know, in detail, what you are going to eat. It is essential that you plan your meals carefully so that you do not unwittingly eat any of the test food.

You may have read about other elimination diets that involve periods of fasting or insist that you stop drinking tea and coffee and stop smoking. The approach outlined in this book asks that all you do is eat your newly simplified diet and eliminate only the food, in all its forms, that you are testing. If you try to eliminate other foods or drinks or try stop smoking at the same time you will make it virtually impossible for yourself to identify what substance is causing what problem.

One food or food chemical at a time.

Elimination diets that ask you to remove a range of foods at one time may, at first, seem like the easiest and most straightforward option. Although avoiding a host of foods at one time may in fact be just as easy as avoiding one, the difficulties arise at the time of testing. Reactions can be delayed and confusing and tests may need to be repeated.

It is also possible to misread results as a study by Bethune et al showed. They reported on how three individuals had self-diagnosed a carbohydrate intolerance and had gone on to develop increasingly restrictive diets as their symptoms kept on reappearing. They found that carbohydrate restriction can disturb glucose metabolism and that this may be interpreted falsely as food allergy.[32] Mumby confirms this and advises against remaining on a very low carbohydrate diet for too long. Although these type of diets can help correct low blood sugar problems they can then go on to reproduce the symptoms if the body is not able to convert sufficient protein into carbohydrate.[33]

These type of blood sugar problems can cause a variety of symptoms many of which mimic allergy problems as well as sometimes being caused by them. These include cravings for sweet foods, feeling tired, anxiety, shaking and inner trembling, depression, irritability, difficulty concentrating, light-headedness, and joint pain. If eating relieves the symptoms at least temporarily then you are likely to have a low blood sugar problem. It is not just eating too little carbohydrate that can cause this it can be that you are simply not eating enough—a risk for anyone changing diets especially if you are keen to lose weight. Make sure that you are eating enough and regularly. Don't worry about the calories as, once your diet settles into one which works for you, the excess weight will gradually fade away without you having to make any effort.

Make sure you check all the labels of any food or drink you are going to consume to ensure it is free of the test food. Eating out could cause problems so phone ahead to the restaurant to see if they can cater for you. Take "safe" snacks with you whenever you go out just in case you need them. It is horrendously frustrating to find yourself needing to eat and not being able to find something that is okay—you are left with the option of potentially making yourself ill or running the risk of low blood sugar problems. It is not a comfortable place to be in.

The length of time that any food or food chemical needs to be eliminated from the diet varies. Generally, for a single food, four to seven days is a reasonable guide. To reduce the impact of a food chemical you need at least seven days, preferably ten to fourteen.

If you have been reacting to the food you have eliminated you can expect a sudden weight loss. This is linked with fluid retention. Breneman found that it is possible to retain as much as 4% of your body weight as fluid as a result of a food sensitivity. This weight is gained within six to eight hours after ingestion and lost within eighteen to twenty four hours after the food has been removed from the diet.[34] You could also find yourself with a headache and feel tired. This is the body detoxifying itself and nothing to worry about. Drink lots of water and rest as much as you can. You may find you suddenly feel amazing and then just as suddenly feel wretched—again this is just detoxification.

And of course, you could just start feeling much better. Be meticulous about keeping your food diary and you will be able to track your progress over time.

Step 6: Test suspect foods

You have now gone the required number of days without eating the test food and the time has come to find out if you have a problem. One very clear indicator is that you have had a noticeable improvement in your symptoms. If this is the case you may want to delay testing for a few more days to ascertain the extent of the "recovery".

Use the strategy agreed with your doctor—this may involve medically supervised allergy tests. If you have been advised to simply reintroduce the food but the change in your symptoms has been dramatic it is best that you recheck with your doctor before testing the food.

If you are testing a single food then choose the time at which you test with care. If you have a busy day planned you do not want to be dealing with unpleasant symptoms at the start of the day.

Eat a reasonable amount of the test food in its simplest most natural form and wait. Some reactions occur immediately or within the first thirty minutes. Common responses are mild swelling in the mouth, headache, feeling disorientated, stomach irritation, a feeling of heaviness and/or lethargy. If you have any of these responses do not continue with the test. You have an intolerance problem to that food.

If nothing happens then continue with your day and note any changes as they occur. Leave at least a few hours before eating any more of the test food. Delayed responses are not uncommon and include a return of your previous symptoms, skin rashes, blood sugar problems, and bloating (hands, feet, abdomen, face, as well as more generally). Reactions can be delayed for as much as thirty six hours.

Testing for a sensitivity to a food chemical is a little more complicated as unwanted reactions tend to occur only after your individual tolerance level has been exceeded. You will need to resume eating foods that have higher amounts of the chemical and carefully note your symptoms over a few days.

Do not attempt to eliminate/test any other food for at least five days. You need to give yourself this amount of time to be sure there is no problem. If after this time you have not experienced any unwanted symptoms then you can assume that the test food is safe. If the test has been inconclusive then you may need to repeat it. Other factors such as illness do have an effect and need to be taken into account. You should also know that it is quite possible to tolerate a food in one form but not another. For example: boiled eggs may be okay but not fried, raw cabbage may make you feel ill but when cooked there is no problem, beef steak may be okay but beef mince could leave you feeling uncomfortable, milk in yoghurt may lead to no symptoms whilst milk on its own causes problems. Test the food in its various forms to be sure you are not unnecessarily eliminating foods from your diet.

Step 7: Review

Was the test food a problem or not? If it was a problem then eliminate it from your diet—you can always retest later. If it wasn't a problem then you can include it in your diet but remember to keep it simple if you are planning further tests. If you have found yourself getting confused then eliminate the test food again and eat your simplified diet for a few days before testing again.

Decide on whether to continue with another test and plan accordingly. Repeat steps 5 to 7 as often as you need and over as long a time period as is appropriate to you.

If your problems continue to remain after food testing then you may like to consider checking your environment for other possible causes—it is not uncommon to react to fragrances and chemicals commonly found in the home, school or work place. Again this is a very hidden problem and only comes to light after you have removed the offending chemical from your environment. It may also be worth exploring whether you have a nutritional deficiency of some sort as these have also been linked with a wide range of conditions and symptoms.

References

[1] Tarlo SM, Sussman GL. Asthma and anaphylactoid reactions to food additives. Can Fam Physician. 1993 May;39:1119-23.

[2] Hawkins CA, Katelaris CH. Nitrate anaphylaxis. Ann Allergy Asthma Immunol. 2000 Jul;85(1):74-6.

[3] Soutter V, Swain A, Loblay, R. Food allergy and food intolerance in young children. Asia Pacific Journal of Clinical Nutrition 1995;4(3):329.

[4] Vatn MH. Food intolerance and psychosomatic experience. Scand J Work Environ Health 1997;23 Suppl 3:75-8.

[5] Hoj L. Diagnostic value of ALCAT test in intolerance to food additives compared with double-blind placebo-controlled (DBPC) oral challenges. Presented at the 52nd Annual Meeting of the American Academy of Allergy, Asthma and Immunology, March 15-20, 1996, New Orleans.

[6] Fell PJ, Brostoff J, O'Donnell H, et al. ALCAT - "a new test for food induced problems in medicine?" Presented at the Annual Meeting of the American Academy of Otolaryngic Allergy, October 1, 1988, Washington, D.C.

[7] Miller JB. A double-blind study of food extract injection therapy: a preliminary report. Ann Allergy 1977;38:185-191.

[8] Lehman CW. A double-blind study of sublingual provocative food testing: a study of its efficacy. Ann Allergy 1980;45:144-149.

[9] Kleine-Tebbe J, Reese I, Ballmer-Weber BK, Beyer K, Erdmann S, et al. No recommendation for IgG and IgG4 testing against foods. Allergo J 2009;4: 267.

[10] Joneja JM. Food Allergy Testing: Problems in Identification of Allergenic Foods. Can J Diet Pract Res 1999;60(4):222-230.

[11] Kim TE, Park SW, Noh GW, Lee SS. Comparison of Skin Prick Test Results between Crude Allergen Extracts from Foods and Commercial Allergen Extracts in Atopic Dermatitis by Double-Blind Placebo-Controlled Food Challenge for Milk, Egg, and Soybean. Yonsei Medical Journal 2002: 43(5); 613-620.

[12] Vojdani A. Detection of IgE, IgG, IgA and IgM antibodies against raw and processed food antigens. Nutr Metab (Lond). 2009 May 12;6:22.

[13] Leduc V, Moneret-Vautrin DA, Guerin L, Morisset M, Kanny G. Anaphylaxis to wheat isolates: immunochemical study of a case proved by means of double-blind, placebo-controlled food challenge. J Allergy Clin Immunol. 2003 Apr;111(4):897-9.

[14] Sloper KS, Wadsworth J, Brostoff J. Children with atopic eczema. I: Clinical response to food elimination and subsequent double-blind food challenge. Q J Med 1991;80(292):677-93.

[15] http://www.which.co.uk/news/2008/08/food-allergy-tests-could-risk-your-health-154711/

[16] Soutter V, Swain A, Loblay, R. Food allergy and food intolerance in young children. Asia Pacific Journal of Clinical Nutrition 1995;4(3):329.

[17] MAFF (Ministry of Agriculture, Fisheries and Food). About food additives. Booklet 2 in food sense ser, 1997.

[18] Hannuksela M, Haahtela T. Hypersensitivity reactions to food additives. Allergy 1987;42(80:561-75.

[19] Antico A, Soana R, Clivio L, Baioni R. Irritable colon syndrome in intolerance to food additives. Minerva Dietol Gastroenterol 1989;35(4):219-24.

[20] Leira R, Rodriguez R. Diet and migraine. Rev Neurol 1996;24:534-8.

[21] Novembre E, Dini L, Bernardini R, Resti M, Vierucci A . Unusual reactions to food additives. Pediatr Med Chir 1992;14(1): 39-42.

[22] Rowe KS, Rowe KJ. Synthetic food coloring and behavior: a dose response effect in a double-blind, placebo-controlled, repeated-measures study. J Pediatr 1994;125(5Pt1):691-8.

[23] Kanny G, De Hauteclocque C, Moneret-Vautrin DA Sesame seed and sesame seed oil contain masked allergens of growing importance. Allergy 1996;51(12):952-7.

[24] Ebo DG, Ingelbrecht S, Bridts CH, Stevens WJ. Allergy for cheese: evidence for an IgE-mediated reaction from the natural dye annatto. Allergy 2009 Oct;64(10):1558-1560.

[25] Scurlock AM, Althage KA, Christie L, Burks AW, Jones SM. Anaphylaxis after ingestion of gummy bears. J Allergy Clin Immunol 2002;1(10).

[26] Feingold B, Feingold H. The Feingold cookbook for hyperactive children and others with problems associated with food additives and salicylates. Random House, 1979.

[27] Hanssen M. E for additives. Thorsons 1991.

[28] Simon R A. Adverse reactions to food and drug additives. J Imm All Clinic NA 1996;16(1):137-76.

[29] Rowe KS, Rowe KJ. Synthetic food coloring and behavior: a dose response effect in a double-blind, placebo-controlled, repeated-measures study. J Pediatr 1994;125(5Pt1):691-8.

[30] Mumby K. Food Allergies and Environmental Illness: the complete guide to. 1993 Thorsons.

[31] Tettenborn M. Health Doctors "allergic to truth about food". BBC News on-line Tue Oct 13 1998.

[32] Bethune CA, Gompels MM, Spickett GP. Physiological effects of starvation interpreted as food allergy. BMJ 1999;319:304-305.

[33] Mumby K. Food Allergies and Environmental Illness: the complete guide to. 1993 Thorsons.

[34] Breneman J. Basics of Food Allergy. Charles C Thomas 1978.

4 Food Chemicals

Food chemicals are compounds found in food that either occur naturally or have been added during the manufacturing process.

As plants produce toxins to protect themselves from spoilage and from being eaten by predators, you cannot avoid the naturally occurring chemicals in food. You can avoid food additives but only if you avoid all forms of processed food. A food chemical, natural, or manmade, becomes a problem for some people when it is eaten in large amounts, is eaten on a regular basis, or the body cannot detoxify it due to illness or a deficiency in the metabolic pathways.

The complexity of each individual plant is immense and any one of its constituent chemicals can, potentially, cause problems for someone sensitive to it. Emsley and Fell estimate that there are about half a million natural chemicals in the food we eat.[1] Only a few of these have been identified and even fewer have been tested, analysed and their implications for health understood.

This section of the book looks at some of the natural chemicals, as well as some of the manmade versions which have often been produced to mimic those produced by nature. The information presented is based on the research done to date and will provide you with an overview of the main chemicals that have been identified as causing problems for some. The key factor to understanding how these chemicals can affect you is to understand that they are most likely cumulative in the body and will generally only cause you a problem if you exceed your own individual tolerance level.

Amines

See also *Histamine, Phenylethylamine, Serotonin, Tyramine.*

Amines are naturally occurring chemicals in certain foods which, like salicylates, are cumulative in the body. Over a period of time these can build up in your system causing reactions that mimic allergies. Amines are produced in food as a result of protein breakdown and/or fermentation which means they are often highly concentrated in processed foods.

If you noticed a substantial decrease in your symptoms when you simplified your diet you may want to consider testing to see if you have an amine problem. If you also regularly suffer from constipation then the amine problem could be more pronounced.

Naturally occurring amines are generally thought to act in the body as neurotransmitters and the term "biogenic amines" is now frequently applied to these. These "biogenic" amines include amongst their number—histamine, phenylethylamine, serotonin and tyramine. Each of these is dealt with separately as each has been found to have clearly defined symptoms in certain individuals.[2,3] Some people, however, seem to have a more general sensitivity to amines. Diets low in food chemicals usually include amines in this more general way.

Cooking certain foods, in particular meats, at high temperatures produces a set of amines that were not present before. One group of these is heterocyclic amines (HCAs). More than seventeen different types of HCAs have been found in meat cooked at high temperatures. Stewing, barbecuing and frying appear to produce the most HCAs. Gravies made from meat juices, therefore, also have a high amine content.

The other form of amine produced by cooking is polycyclic aromatic hydrocarbons (PAH). These are formed by the browning of carbohydrate based foods such as bread and are also found in foods such as smoked and grilled meats and coffee. A sensitivity to these amines can often be misinterpreted as an intolerance specific to one type of food. For example, if toast doesn't agree with you it is easy to think that wheat is the problem; if a grilled steak upsets you then you might think you have a problem with beef.

What everybody should know is that various studies have linked these types of amines with cancer. The rule of thumb here is do not overcook food and always eat your food as fresh as possible. Pickling, smoking and other forms of preserving all increase the number of amines.

There is no specific list of symptoms indicated for amines but migraines that don't respond to other treatments may be relieved by a diet low in amines. The key to testing for an amine intolerance is to reduce the amount of amines in your diet, and hence your body, over a period of two weeks. Stick to your simplified diet as much as possible but eliminate all the high amine foods.

Re-think your cooking style. Avoid over cooking anything and avoid meat cooked in sauces as these will have a high amine content. Never eat anything that has been burnt and avoid toasted breakfast cereals. After two weeks, eat some of your most favourite high amine foods and monitor your response. Remember that amines are cumulative in the body.

Some people may immediately get a reaction such as a headache or digestive problems and others will only get similar symptoms after their level has increased—this can take up two weeks so keep your food diary up to date.

At the end of the testing time, if you have felt no better at all then you are unlikely to have an amine problem. If there has been a little improvement you may want to consider reducing your level even further and seeing if that increases the improvement. You should, however, also note that individuals who are intolerant of one chemical in food often are intolerant of another so you may need to test some of the other food chemicals.

If you have had a substantial improvement then you are amine sensitive and need to now work on establishing the level of amines you can generally tolerate. At this stage you may find your tolerance is very low but that over time this may change.

Establishing the amine content of food is quite difficult as it can be greatly affected by the way food is stored, processed and cooked. Avoiding the foods in the list below for a week or two should be enough to give you an idea as to whether you are especially sensitive to amines or not.

Foods high in amines

All forms of processed meats including sausages, pâtés, bacon, salamis, deli counter cuts.

All forms of processed fish including fish cakes and fish fingers.

All smoked, salted and pickled meats and fish.

All offal including kidneys, liver and brains.

Game and other meat that has been "matured".

Cheese (whilst some very mild cheeses may be okay it is easier, at this stage, to avoid them all)

Fermented bean products such as tofu, tempeh, bean curd, miso, soy sauce, tamari.

Pickled vegetables such as sauerkraut, gherkins and piccalillis.

Cocoa, dark chocolate, milk chocolate high in cocoa solids.

Meat extracts, gravies, sauces, yeast extracts.

Chocolate flavoured drinks, cola type drinks, vegetable and fruit juices.

Beer and wine.

Benzoates

See also *Salicylate*.

Benzoic acid occurs naturally in many berries, fruits, herbs and spices (such as cinnamon and cloves), vegetables and tea. The existence of benzoic acid in its natural form has been known since at least the sixteenth century. The body generally excretes benzoic acid as hippuric acid in the urine within nine to fifteen hours after ingestion but it's presence in the body can temporarily inhibit function of digestive enzymes and may deplete amino acid glycine levels.

In around 1860 it was produced synthetically from compounds derived from coal tar. Today, one of the ways it is commercially manufactured is by the chemical reaction of toluene, a hydrocarbon obtained from petroleum, with oxygen in the presence of cobalt and manganese salts as catalysts.

The commercial form is used in the food manufacturing process as a preservative and also has widespread non-food uses. The use of derivatives such as benzoyl peroxide for bleaching flour (at the time of writing, not allowed in the UK) is an example of how this can become a hidden sensitivity as bleaching agents rarely have to be declared on products they have been used in. The intakes from natural sources are low in comparison with potential intakes from food additive uses. Symptoms of benzoate sensitivity have included:

Angioedema, Asthma aggravation, Gastrointestinal problems, Hyperactivity, Itching, Numbing effect in the mouth, Recurrent urticaria, Rhinitis, Skin sensitivity.

Jacobsen writes that people with asthma, chronic urticaria-angioedema, rhinitis, and purpura may be predisposed towards benzoate and paraben sensitivity.[4] Wuthrich and Fabro found benzoate sensitivity in some individuals suffering from asthma, rhinitis, and urticaria.[5] Juhlin et al examined the sensitivity of aspirin-intolerant people to p-hydroxybenzoate and sodium benzoate by oral provocation testing; urticaria was induced in five of seven people.[6]

Michaelsson and Juhlin's study of fifty seven people with recurrent urticaria or angioedema found that 52% reacted to sodium benzoate and/or p-hydroxybenzoic acid.[7] August reported that thirty three out of eighty six people with chronic urticaria gave positive reactions to tartrazine and sodium benzoate.[8] Gibson and Chancy found that 52% of people studied with chronic idiopathic urticaria had a benzoate sensitivity.[9]

Ortolani et al found 21% of a patient group with chronic urticaria-angioedema were intolerant to benzoic acid. They also noted a high incidence of cross-reactivity to aspirin.[10] Chafee and Settipane found that sodium benzoate might have been responsible for the provocation of asthma in a patient who had taken a dye-free vitamin supplement preserved with benzoate. Investigations showed a sensitivity to tartrazine; the reaction to the supplement could have been due to the fact that tartrazine and benzoates have the same aromatic ring structure and carbohydrate group and hence are viewed as virtually the same by the body.[11]

Asero wrote about the case of a seventy-five year old woman who, for six years, had suffered from severe itching but with no evidence of a rash. She had been treated with various anti-histamines but none had resolved the problem. Various skin prick tests were carried out but all were negative. After following an elimination diet for ten days, the itching had reduced in severity by 80% and had totally disappeared a week later. Further tests were carried out and it was discovered that the culprit was sodium benzoate.[12] Reactions to this group of additives have been observed in people with an aspirin or salicylate sensitivity and should be avoided by anyone with this condition.

If you suspect a problem with benzoates, the food additives you need to avoid are:

E210 Benzoic acid
E211 Sodium benzoate
E212 Potassium benzoate
E213 Calcium benzoate
E214 Ethyl p-hydroxybenzoate
E215 Sodium ethyl p-hydroxybenzoate
E218 Methyl p-hydroxybenzoate
E219 Sodium methyl p-hydroxybenzoate

You may also need to limit your intake of foods in which benzoates occur naturally. Now this is not totally straightforward as, just like with amines and some other naturally occurring food chemicals, there is no definitive list for benzoate levels in food. It is generally thought that high levels occur in the following:[13]

Most fruit berries but especially strawberries and raspberries.

Tea.

Herbs and spices especially anise, cinnamon, clove, nutmeg, and thyme.

Condiments such as soy sauce.

If you suspect benzoates are causing you a problem then eliminate them as best as you can from your diet for at least two weeks. If there are signs of improvement then continue to avoid them for a further two weeks before testing. Partial improvement with a reaction after testing could indicate that you need to check non-food substances for benzoates and also avoid these but if this does not work then testing for a salicylate sensitivity is probably indicated as both salicylates and benzoates have similar chemical structures.

Esters of para-hydroxybenzoic acid, more commonly known as parabens, are used widely in medications and cosmetics. In fact, benzoates can be found in a variety of non-food products including medicines, perfumes, cosmetics, toothpaste, lice treatments, resin preparations, in the production of plasticisers, in dyestuffs, synthetic fibres, as a chemical intermediate, as a corrosion inhibitor in paints, a curing agent in tobacco, as a mordant in calico printing and in insecticides. Some exposure may also result from inhalation of auto exhaust, tobacco smoke and other combustion sources.

Caffeine

Caffeine is one of three dietary methylxanthines, the other two being theobromine and theophylline. All three are readily absorbed from the gastrointestinal tract and distributed throughout the body, metabolised in the liver and excreted in the urine. Theobromine is weak in comparison to caffeine, and theophylline is only found in small concentrations in food so the only methylxanthine dealt with in this book is caffeine.

Caffeine naturally occurs in the leaves, seeds or fruits of at least sixty three plant species world-wide. The most familiar sources of caffeine in our diet are through drinks such as coffee, tea and cola. The amount of caffeine in any product varies depending on the plant variety used and also how it was prepared.

Caffeine is so readily available in coffee, tea and chocolate that we have come to accept it as harmless but the truth is that caffeine is a powerful drug that affects both your body and your mind. It has the strange quality of at first decreasing the heart rate and then increasing it about an hour after intake. It, also, has a powerful effect on the nervous system and can, in small doses, help improve concentration but the reverse takes place with a higher dose.

Even a relatively moderate amount, two to three cups of tea a day, leads to observable effects and caffeine abuse can result in symptoms that mimic mental illness. Children, because they have smaller bodies, are at greater risk from caffeine toxicity, and insomnia in children could be linked to the amount of cola drinks they consume.[14,15] How much caffeine you can tolerate will depend on a number of factors including the amount you consume, how often you consume it, and your individual metabolism.

Some people seem to experience no noticeable effects whilst others have uncomfortable symptoms after just a small amount. Products containing caffeine are often used to boost energy which takes place as a result of caffeine's ability to stimulate adrenal gland activity. This constant abuse of the adrenal glands can, however, lead to a state of burn out where the adrenal glands quite simply become exhausted. Fatigue, although it can have many causes, can often be the result of diminished adrenal function. If this is the case, no amount of additional coffee or chocolate will help.

The speed at which your body is able to eliminate caffeine depends on factors such as age, state of health and your own unique biochemical make-up. The rate at which it is cleared is decreased by liver disease, pregnancy and oral contraceptives. Women taking oral contraceptives have been found to have significantly lower rates for breaking down caffeine than women not using these contraceptives and men.[16]

Fluoroquinolines, drugs used to treat bacterial infections, impair caffeine and theophylline metabolism leading to a greater concentration in the body.[17] Other medications, including theophylline, can also cause a problem as these can add to the stimulant effects of caffeine-containing foods and drinks.

Sadly, caffeine is habit forming and tolerance develops so that more and more is required to obtain the desired effect. Silverman et al found that even consuming smaller regular doses of caffeine can lead to addiction.[18] A variety of conditions have been linked with a caffeine sensitivity. Charney et al, in a placebo controlled study of people with panic disorder or agoraphobia with panic attacks found that caffeine significantly increases anxiety, nervousness, fear, nausea, palpitations, restlessness and tremors. These effects all correlated with plasma caffeine levels.[19]

Observations made by Davis and Osorio suggest that caffeine may precipitate tics in susceptible children.[20] Greden found that caffeine in large quantities of tea and coffee could produce symptoms that mimic anxiety and panic disorders.[21] Even caffeine induced urticaria has been noted.[22,23] In one case a sixteen year old woman had experienced episodes of generalised urticaria for about eight years. They appeared to be linked with ingestion of cola drinks. The episodes had at times been severe enough to require emergency treatment. Various ingredients were tested using the skin prick test but were all negative. A double blind, placebo-controlled, oral challenge test, was performed with a regular cola drink and a decaffeinated cola-drink. The regular cola-drink provoked itching and urticaria on her body and legs within ten minutes. The caffeine-free cola-drink elicited no adverse reactions. A skin prick test confirmed that caffeine was the trigger.[24]

The symptoms that have been linked to a caffeine sensitivity or to a high intake of caffeine include:

> Agitation, Anxiety, Blood Sugar Problems, Depression, Disorientation, Dry mouth, Headache, Heartburn, Increased need to urinate, Insomnia, Irritability, Nausea, Palpitations, Panic Attacks, Restless legs syndrome, Rhinitis, Stomach problems, Sweating, Tinnitus, Tremors, Urticaria.

It is quite possible that regular headaches or migraines are linked with caffeine withdrawal. If you have any of the above symptoms and consume large amounts of caffeine then consider testing for caffeine sensitivity. The only way of assessing sensitivity is to eliminate all caffeine from the diet for ten days, reassess the situation and then reintroduce it if you choose too. If you consume large amounts of caffeine and are concerned about the effect of withdrawal symptoms then reduce the amount that you use over a period of ten days until you are as caffeine free as you can manage. Make a list of how much caffeine you consume and draw up a reducing strategy. Choose the best option for you. The foods you need to eliminate/reduce are all forms of:

Coffee, tea, chocolate and cocoa, cola drinks, guarana, mate and any other soft drinks that contain caffeine.

To be on the safe side also check any medications, supplements and tonics. Any prescribed forms of medication containing caffeine should be continued until you have discussed them with your doctor and been given permission to reduce or stop taking them.

You will either find that you very quickly begin to feel calmer and less stressed or will begin to experience withdrawal symptoms. Do not be alarmed if you find yourself feeling ill. All of the following have been linked with caffeine withdrawal: low attention span, depression, nervousness, problems sleeping, mood swings, and irritability. Drink lots of water and be gentle with yourself and let your body do the job of detoxification.

The positive changes you are looking for are an increase in energy but less manic, fewer sleeping problems, increased ability to concentrate, more relaxed, less irritable and nervous, and a peaceful sense of well being. If you experience any of the above then you really should question the sense of returning to using any products containing caffeine.

Replacements in the form of decaffeinated coffee and tea, caffeine free drinks and carob bars are all now readily available and make acceptable substitutes. If you do return to using caffeine products ensure you keep them to a minimum in your diet—if you don't then before you know it all the symptoms will have returned. For example, some people may get away with two cups of coffee and a bar of chocolate, or three cups of tea, or two cans of cola and some may not be able to tolerate any at all.

If you have gone through withdrawal then the safest course of action is to quite simply say NO to caffeine. This also applies to anyone that has or is suffering from anxiety or depression as the intensity of both of these states can be exacerbated by caffeine.

The amount of caffeine in various products is a matter of some dispute. For example, some studies show no caffeine in chocolate, others have shown a large amount. As caffeine has definitely been found in chocolate and cocoa it is safest to eliminate it at this time. Also please note that even decaffeinated drinks may still contain some caffeine albeit in small amounts.

One example of estimated amounts of caffeine in products comes from a UK survey:[25]

Non decaffeinated cola drinks	33 to 213 mg/l
Low caffeine colas	less than 0.2 mg/l
Energy drinks	0.5 to 349 mg/l
Standard tea products	95 to 430 mg/l
Instant and ground coffee	105 to 340 mg/l
Decaffeinated instant coffee	10 to 11 mg/l
Chocolate products	5.5 to 710 mg/kg
(highest levels in chocolate bars)	

Be cautious if your caffeine intake is mainly from cola drinks and your preference is for the diet free variety as these tend to be higher in caffeine than full sugar colas.[26]

Rozin et al found that a chocolate bar contains 20mg of caffeine compared to 80-100mg in a cup of coffee. This relatively low dose in comparison with other sources of caffeine, such as coffee and cola drinks, which are not craved to the same extent, suggests that caffeine is not the major reason that chocolate is craved. However, if you are extremely sensitive to caffeine it could be a problem.[27]

Capsaicin

The genus "capsicum" encompasses several species including chilli peppers, red peppers, and paprika. Capsaicin is the most important biologically active compound within these and it is known for providing pain relief in conditions such as arthritis and neuralgia. It can also have an adverse effect if you are sensitive to it.

The most common adverse reaction is a burning sensation in the mouth but others have also been noted. Serio et al outline a case of plasma cell gingivitis linked with exposure to capsaicin.[28] Myers et al found it led to a significant increase in gastric acid secretion as well as mucosal bleeding.[29] Evidence of nausea, vomiting and abdominal pain after ingestion have also been noted, and exposure in the workplace has led to cases of coughs being linked with its inhalation and to contact dermatitis.

To test for a sensitivity eliminate all of the following from your diet for at least five days:

> Bell pepper, cayenne, cherry pepper, chilli, cone pepper, green pepper, hot pepper, paprika, red chilli, spur pepper, sweet pepper, tabasco.

Be very careful with any pre-prepared meals and sauces or restaurant food as some of these may contain capsaicin under the term "spices". After the elimination period, test by eating whichever one you used to eat most often in as simple a form as possible. If you get a reaction then wait another five days before trying a different food from the list.

The reason for testing more than one is to ensure that the problems you are experiencing stem from capsaicin and not the individual food. If you experience no reaction then capsaicin is unlikely to be a problem for you.

Gluten

See also: *Grains, Wheat.*

Gluten is made up of a number of proteins including gliadin and naturally occurs in a number of grains.

Gluten has been linked with a number of conditions most notably dermatitis herpetiformis and coeliac disease. Atherton states that there can be no real doubt that dietary gluten is responsible for most, if not all dermatitis herpetiformis.[30] Feighery writes that coeliac disease is an inflammatory disease of the upper small intestine and results from gluten ingestion in genetically susceptible individuals. Treatment consists of permanent withdrawal of gluten from the diet resulting in complete remission.[31]

Other conditions have also been found to be linked with gluten sensitivity. These include Crohn's disease, diabetes, irritable bowel syndrome, and rheumatoid arthritis.[32] In one study, twenty individuals who had suffered from recurrent aphthous ulcers, some for more than eleven years, were given a gluten-free diet to follow. Five of these became ulcer free and when challenge tested with gluten the ulcers returned.[33]

Mental symptoms that respond to no other treatment may also benefit from a gluten-free diet. In the book *Brain Allergies*, Philpott and Kalita note that "After years of observing maladaptive mental reactions to foods, most orthomolecular-ecologic psychiatrists would agree that gluten is the most frequent and severe symptom reactor of all foods".[34]

Braly and Hoggan explore the links that have been found between gluten sensitivity and various "brain disorders" including ADHD, autism, depression, epilepsy, multiple sclerosis, schizophrenia, senility, and sleeping problems. Whilst links are being found the authors acknowledge that a great deal more research needs to be done so that links between brain disorders and diet are taken seriously.[35]

The gluten grains are barley, rye and wheat. Oats are also included and on a gluten-free diet should at least in the first instance be excluded but then tested as some gluten sensitives have found them safe. There are tests available that will establish if you have a gluten sensitivity but you can also exclude gluten from your diet to see if there is any improvement. The difficulty is that if you see an improvement you will not know if it is because of a grain sensitivity (to one or more of those excluded) or a gluten intolerance. Given this difficulty you would be advised to test the grains individually over a period of time to ensure that you are clear about what it is that is causing you problems, this will help prevent you limiting your diet unnecessarily.

If you need to eat a gluten-free diet you will need to avoid all foods that contain wheat (including spelt, triticale and kamut), rye, barley and possibly oats. Alternatives will need to be found for bread, cakes, pastries and biscuits. It is also essential that you check all processed foods, including meats, to avoid accidental ingestion.

Although oats are often excluded on a gluten-free diet there is increasing amounts of evidence that they are in fact tolerated by many individuals with a measurable gluten sensitivity; it is also now possible to buy oats that are certified as being gluten free. Janatuninen et al, in a study of adults with coeliac disease, compared the effects of a gluten-free diet including oats with a conventional gluten-free diet. They concluded that adults with coeliac disease can consume moderate amounts of oats without adverse immunological effects.[36]

Hallert et al carried out a review of published reports in 1999 and also presented details of their own experience at including oats in the gluten-free diets of adults. They found oats to be safe and well tolerated by adults with coeliac disease and dermatitis herpetiformis, though the risk of wheat contamination of commercial oat products was a cause of concern.[37]

Reunala et al carried out a study to ascertain the tolerance to oats by individuals with dermatitis herpetiformis. Eleven individuals on gluten-free diets with the condition were challenged daily with 50g oats for six months. A control group comprised of eleven people with dermatitis herpetiformis on a conventional gluten-free diet were also studied. Eight of those challenged with oats remained symptom free, two developed a transient rash, and one withdrew because of the appearance of a more persistent but mild rash. It should be noted that three of the eleven controls also developed a transient rash. Various tests were conducted to measure the impact, if any, of the oats, and the conclusions were that oats do not affect gluten sensitive small bowel mucosa and indicate that dermatitis herpetiformis is not activated by eating oats.[38]

Given this evidence the wisest course may be to, at first, exclude oats along with the other grains and then, once the condition has been stabilised, to test oats but only those classed as gluten-free.

Although gluten is now seen as the cause of coeliac disease this was not always the case. As Gottschall tells us, prior to 1952, coeliac disease was being treated as a carbohydrate intolerance problem by a specific carbohydrate avoidance diet. She argues that the gluten-free diet does not work for all sufferers because of the continued use of carbohydrates. It is certainly the case that straightforward avoidance of gluten does not work for everyone.[39]

It cannot be disputed that gluten-free diets help many people but the reality is that for some individuals with dermatitis herpetiformis and/or coeliac disease removal of gluten is not the answer or at least not the whole answer. A study by Faulkner-Hogg et al found that some individuals with coeliac disease who did not wholly improve on a gluten-free diet were sensitive to salicylate. On testing, salicylate was found to provoke diarrhoea, headache, nausea and flatulence.[40]

Braly and Hoggan recognised that some coeliac patients continued to have symptoms even after following a strict gluten-free diet. Their symptoms improved or disappeared when their other food sensitivities were identified. The most common problem foods were found to be milk, soy, corn, egg, citrus fruit, and seafood.[41]

An Australian study set out to explore why some people with coeliac disease continue to have symptoms even when following a gluten-free diet. Thirty nine adults who had persistent gastrointestinal symptoms despite adhering to a gluten-free diet were evaluated. They discovered that twenty two were consuming a gluten-free diet as defined by the WHO/FAO Codex Alimentarius (Codex-GFD) in which foods containing up to 0.3% of protein from gluten-containing grains can be labelled as "gluten free". The remaining seventeen were following a "no detectable gluten diet" as defined by Food Standards, Australia.

All thirty nine followed the "no detectable gluten diet" during the study. For five, of the twenty two who made the change in diet, symptoms disappeared and were reduced for a further ten. Food elimination diets were then tried with thirty-one of the participants leading to further improvement for twenty four of them. The three most common problems were soya, amines and salicylates. They argue that if symptoms persist after following a "no detectable gluten diet" then other food sensitivities should be explored.[42]

The way food is labelled varies from country to country. In the UK, January 2012 saw the introduction of new rules on how food can be labelled with claims about gluten. The law covers all food, whether it is in a packet on a supermarket shelf, on a menu in a restaurant, or at a deli counter. This means that any food making claims about gluten content has to stick to strict low levels. These rules mean that food can be labelled as:

Gluten-free—these foods are suitable for people with coeliac disease (they can have no more than 20 parts of gluten per million).

Very low gluten— small amounts of these foods can be eaten by most coeliacs, but they should get advice from a dietitian or health professional about how often they can eat them. (These foods must contain no more than 100 parts of gluten per million, and must contain ingredients that have been specially processed to reduce their gluten content, so this labelling will be mostly found on specialist products).

The phrase **"suitable for coeliacs"**, can only be used alongside the terms "gluten-free" or "very low gluten" and can't be used on its own.[43]

To avoid gluten you need to very carefully check the ingredients of all foods. Some of the terms that might indicate the presence of gluten include:

Baking powder, barley, barley grass, barley malt, beer, blue cheese, bran, bread, bulgar, caramel, cereal, couscous, dextrins, durum, farina, flour, groats, gum, HPP (hydrolyzed plant protein), HVP (hydrolyzed vegetable protein), kamut, malt, matzo, miso, MSG (monosodium glutamate), mustard powder, oats, pearl barley, rice malt, rye, semolina, soy sauce, spelt, starch, stock cubes, teriyaki sauce, TPP (textured plant protein), triticale, TVP (textured vegetable protein),wheat, wheatgerm.

The addictive nature of some foods and food chemicals is not something that there is general agreement about yet it is something that undeniably exists. One of the difficulties seems to be when a food, or aspect of a food like gluten, is reduced in the diet but not fully eliminated and this constant small amount in the body seems to lead to cravings for products that contain the food or food chemical. Braly and Hoggan make specific reference to the addictive nature of gluten and the problems this causes some individuals when first attempting to eat a gluten free diet.[44]

The same authors also note that a powerful tobacco addiction can indicate a sensitivity to gluten. They write that smoking "can amount to a form of neurochemical 'self-medication' for those who have problems with gluten". For individuals affected in this way, attempting to stop smoking before they have dealt with their gluten problem can lead to depression and mood disturbances.

Histamine

See also *Amines.*

Histamine is a biogenic amine that occurs in many different foods. At extremely high concentrations, usually as a result of food spoilage, it can lead to poisoning. In some individuals smaller concentrations can lead to food intolerance which is often misinterpreted and can lead to the wrong food being eliminated.

The problems associated with an overload of histamine were first recorded in 1830 when crew members of a vessel became ill with severe headaches, flushing, bloating, diarrhoea and shivering after eating bonito, a member of the Scomberesociade fish family. The illness was called "scombroid poisoning". As other types of fish were also found to cause similar symptoms, research was conducted to find the common link. That common link turned out to be histamine.[45]

Histamine poisoning differs from histamine sensitivity. In cases of histamine poisoning the person is likely to have eaten a contaminated form of fish and experienced a reaction almost immediately. The symptoms, usually a combination of sweating/shivering, rashes, flushing, burning sensation in the mouth, stomach pains, diarrhoea and headache, last for about twelve hours and then abate.

Histamine sensitivity is unlikely to result in such severe symptoms and may not abate as quickly. The body already has a supply of histamine which it stores in a safe form for use when needed. Food too high in histamine swamps the body's defences. If the body becomes flooded with histamine in a "non-safe" form problems can arise. The body has to act to clear it and fast and in some individuals this clearance mechanism is slow and, whenever their tolerance level is breached, unwanted symptoms arise.[46]

The suspected cause is a deficiency of diamine oxidase in the small intestine resulting in diminished histamine degradation in the gastrointestinal tract, and thus absorption.[47] A sensitivity to histamine can produce allergy type symptoms which no allergy test will recognise. Histamine is heat stable—cooking does not remove it.

Wantke's study in 1993 found that sensitivity to histamine in food and drink could result in bronchial asthma, headache, and urticaria. He also found the ingestion of food rich in histamine brought about a recurrence of atopic eczema in those affected.[48] Doeglas et al identified histamine intoxication after eating cheese in some individuals; the symptoms included nausea, vomiting, urticaria, headache, difficulty swallowing and thirst.[49]

Ingestion of 25 to 50mg of histamine can trigger headaches, and 100-150mg can lead to flushing.[50] However, figures such as these can only ever be estimates. Scombroid toxicity has been identified after ingestion of only 2.5mg of histamine.[51]

Histamine sensitivity can lead to a range of symptoms including:

Abdominal cramps, Angioedema, Asthma like symptoms, Bronchial asthma, Burning sensation in the mouth and throat, Conjunctivitis, Diarrhoea, Difficulty swallowing, Dizziness, Eczema, Flushing, Headaches, Low blood pressure, Migraines, Nausea and vomiting, Palpitations, Peppery taste in the mouth, Rhinitis, Shortness of breath, Skin itching, Sneezing, Urticaria.

Testing for a histamine sensitivity is advisable in cases of chronic headaches, migraines and skin complaints that don't respond to other solutions. A common indicator of a histamine problem is if you know that red wine always gives you a headache. The key to testing for histamine sensitivity is to ensure you eat your food as fresh as possible. Then totally avoid all the foods on the list below. As so many cheeses are implicated I would suggest that you avoid all cheese for the duration of the test which should be at least seven days.

After seven clear days eat a meal containing one of the foods on the list that you would ordinarily eat (not cheese) and monitor your reaction. If you have unpleasant symptoms within a few hours you would be advised to avoid foods high in histamine. If you have no problems then you can gradually reintroduce the foods but keep a food diary and monitor your progress—it could be that you can tolerate a reasonable amount but not too much. When you are secure in establishing your tolerance then reintroduce cheese (not one of those listed).

The reason for postponing the testing of cheese is that it is possible to have a hidden milk sensitivity and this would cloud the results of the histamine test. Should you find that you have a problem with a cheese not on this list I recommend that you test for milk intolerance.

More detailed information on histamine content of food is difficult to come by as measurement is not a straightforward process due to variations in food affected by factors such as storage and fermentation. The list below, compiled from various sources including Joneja[52] and Maintz[53], is, therefore, not a definitive list and the amounts of histamine in foods included will vary considerably'

Fish: Anchovy, herring, mackerel, sardine, salmon, tuna.

Cheese: Blue, camembert, cheddar, emmental, gouda, harzer, mozzarella, parmesan, provolone, roquefort, swiss, tilsiter.

Meat: All dried or cured meats such as hams and salamis.

Vegetables: Aubergine, sauerkraut, spinach, tomatoes.

Alcohol: Beer, champagne, red wine, sparkling wine, white wine.

Other: Tamari, soy sauce, tomato ketchup.

More generally avoid any food that has been smoked, pickled or fermented.

You will need to use a food diary to monitor your responses. Some foods without a significant histamine content have been thought to trigger a histamine release.[54] Foods with this capacity include:

Egg white, crustaceans, chocolate, strawberries, tomatoes and citrus fruit.

How long the effects of histamine will last depends upon its metabolism in the body. Under "normal" circumstances, histamine is rapidly converted to its inactive metabolites by either histamine methyltransferase or diamine oxidase (DAO).[55] It has also been found that eating a histamine containing meal and taking drugs that inhibit DAO can produce symptoms so check with your doctor about any medication that you are taking.

Once you have established your level of histamine tolerance, adjust your diet to accommodate it. You will need to ensure that you never eat too many foods high in histamine in succession but if you are able to tolerate some you will be to included these in your weekly meal plan. Histamine-intolerant women often suffer from headaches that are dependent on their menstrual cycle and from dysmenorrhoea.[56]

Lectins

See also *Legumes.*

Lectins are a class of proteins, chiefly of plant origin, which bind specifically to certain sugars and cause agglutination of particular cell types. It has now been found that lectins are toxic and/or inflammatory, resistant to cooking and digestive enzymes, and present in much of our food. Initially it was thought that lectins only caused digestive problems that often mimicked the symptoms of food poisoning but it is now believed that some of these leave the gut and affect other organs in the body leading to more widespread symptoms.

Many lectins are powerful allergens in their own right, such as prohevin, the principle allergen of rubber latex, but it is also possible to be more generally sensitive. One of the most commonly known lectins is phytohaemagglutinin which is found in beans.

Gilbert reports on a case of a hospital holding a "healthy eating day" which resulted in illness. The canteen served a dish containing red kidney beans which was chosen by 31 customers. Over the next few hours cases of severe vomiting and diarrhoea were reported. All had recovered by next day. Investigations showed no signs of traditional food poisoning but the beans were found to contain an abnormally high concentration of the lectin phytohaemagglutinin.[57]

Ordinarily, phytohaemagglutinin is only a danger after consumption of raw or undercooked kidney beans. The reactions experienced after eating beans in this state are classed as a form of poisoning not intolerance. In these situations, the symptoms usually appear within one to three hours and are marked by extreme nausea, followed by vomiting, abdominal pain and diarrhoea. Some people have been hospitalised but recovery is usually rapid.

Phytohaemagglutinin is found in many species of bean but it is found in highest concentrations in the red kidney bean. Soaking the beans reduces the number of lectins but adequate cooking is still required. Whilst white kidney beans have fewer of these lectins, soaking does not reduce the number significantly so they too are not to be eaten raw.[58]

Some people find that, even when cooked correctly, red kidney beans cause problems most notably abdominal discomfort. The only solution is to avoid the beans. Information on testing for a sensitivity to beans can be found in the section on *Legumes*.

The different ways in which we deal with lectins has also been linked with blood groups types.[59] And, reviewing the available research, Freed suggested that it was possible that insulin dependent diabetes, rheumatoid arthritis, and peptic ulcers could all be triggered by problems with lectins. The avoidance of large numbers of lectins in diets such as the "stone age" diet could be the reason why some people notice an improvement in their symptoms especially in reducing respiratory symptoms as without lectins in the throat the lining provides a more effective barrier to viruses.

Freed goes on to offer an explanation as to how disease such as rheumatoid arthritis and diabetes can often develop after illnesses such as flu. Basically, the protective coating of our cells can be stripped away during illness leaving us open to the damaging effect of lectins.[60]

Lectins are increasingly being implicated in auto immune illnesses, coeliac disease, arthritis, and some forms of diabetes. As Hamid and Masood write "The involvement of lectins in our health and their relationship to degenerative disease is still an emerging science".[61] At the moment there are no comprehensive lists regarding types of lectin and levels in food nor is there detailed information on the possible benefits or otherwise of specific lectins.

One of the strongest indicators of a lectin problem is if you develop health issues after changing to a diet high in legumes. I suspect it is also an area to consider if rheumatoid arthritis is not responding to other treatments.

Lectins are found in most plant foods but certain categories of food have been identified as causing more problems than others. In a possible order of potential problems, these are given below:

Legumes including peanuts and soy.

Cereal grains especially wheat.

Potatoes and tomatoes and other members of the deadly nightshade family (see the section on *Solanine*).

If you suspect a problem with lectins the best place to start would be with removing legumes from the diet. If there is a problem, symptoms should begin to disappear within a few days.

Establishing detailed information on lectin content of plant foods is not straightforward—not all plants have been tested, tests have been done in different ways, and we still do not know which lectins are beneficial. A study by Ramona et al found lectin concentration HU/mg in the sixteen foods analysed as follows:[62]

Red kidney beans 360
Red lentils 360
Chick peas 180
Pinto beans 180
Soya beans 87
Black eyed peas 44
Porridge Oats 17
Banana 13
All bran cereal 5.6
Digestive biscuits 5.6
Potato 5.5
White rice, wholemeal bread, white spaghetti all had less than 1.3.

In respect of grains, lectin activity has been found in wheat, rye, barley, oats, corn and rice but not in millet or sorghum.[63]

MSG

MSG, monosodium glutamate, is the sodium salt of a naturally occurring amino acid—glutamic acid. Glutamate is essential to life and is found in cells throughout our body. It occurs in two forms, naturally in food and as an added flavour enhancer. Most of the glutamate our bodies receive is in a "bound" form and is gradually released as enzymes digest the protein food that it is part of. MSG, on the other hand, is a form of "free" glutamate that is instantly available to us and it is too much of this type that can lead to problems.

The degree of sensitivity experienced depends on the individual. Some people can tolerate vast amounts, others find themselves shaking and in an anxiety state after very little. The "toxic" reactions experienced by some people are generally because of an overload of MSG in its form as a flavour enhancer.

MSG intensifies some flavours and lessens others. It is an ideal additive for food manufacturers to "adjust" the taste of highly processed food and you can, without realising it, be ingesting quite large amounts of MSG. Generally made from the fermentation of corn, sugar beets, or sugar cane, MSG is a potential problem for anyone with an intolerance of these foods.

MSG has been linked with a number of conditions. It has been found to bring on asthma in some individuals, with the asthma developing anywhere from one to two hours to as long as twelve hours after ingestion.[64,65] More general concerns have been expressed about damage being caused to the nervous system and brain cells which can contribute to the onset of serious illnesses, like Parkinson's disease and dementia, in later life.[66]

Squire reported on a case of a fifty-year old man whose recurrent angioedema of the face, hands and feet was related to MSG intake. The angioedema occurred sixteen to twenty four hours after ingestion of MSG.[67] Botey et al reported on four children whose urticaria was caused by MSG. Symptoms developed between one and twelve hours after the MSG challenge was given.[68]

A condition that became known as "Chinese Restaurant Syndrome" was identified in the late 1960s and linked MSG with a collection of symptoms including headaches, stomach pains, breathing problems, nausea and thirst.[69]

In summary, the various symptoms and conditions that have been linked with MSG sensitivity are listed below. These have been combined from a number of sources including the review in Joneja's book[70].

> Anxiety, Asthma, Balance problems, Behavioural problems, Bloating, Blood pressure changes, Blurred vision, Breathing difficulties, Burning sensation in the back of the neck and forearms, Changes in heart rate, Chest pain, Depression, Diarrhoea, Difficulty focusing, Disorientation, Dizziness, Extreme dryness of the mouth, Facial tightness, Flu-like achiness, Flushing, Headache, Hyperactivity, Insomnia, Irritable bowel, Joint pain, Lethargy, Light-headedness, Loss of balance, Mental confusion, Migraine, Mood Swings, Nausea, Numbness or paralysis, Panic attacks, Paranoia, Rapid heartbeat, Runny nose, Sciatica, Seizures, Shortness of breath, Skin rashes, Sleepiness, Slurred speech, Stiffness, Stomach cramps, Urinary and prostate problems, Wheezing.

Fatigue has been noted as a side effect of too much MSG. As this often occurs up to twelve hours after ingesting MSG it is sometimes difficult to link the symptoms to the cause (a food diary will help). If you frequently eat food containing large amounts of MSG, such as some forms Chinese takeout, then you may have a hidden MSG problem.

MSG does seem to set away an addictive response and hence cause food cravings. One of the difficulties with diagnosing if you have an MSG sensitivity is that it is often an ingredient that is hidden. You will need to follow the avoidance process very carefully.

To test for MSG sensitivity avoid all foods containing added MSG for at least five days. Avoid the additives:

E621 Monosodium glutamate
E622 Monopotassium glutamate
E623 Calcium diglutamate
E624 Monoammonium glutamate
E625 Magnesium diglutamate

Unfortunately this is not a straightforward process. These additives creep into many foods and it is probably best if during these five days you avoid eating any restaurant or take-out food and preferably only eat what you cook yourself. The foods to check carefully include:

All ready meals.

Snack foods such as cheese and spicy flavoured crisps, chips, tacos.

Soya products, mainly soy sauce, miso, tamari, tempeh.

Most sauces, gravy mixes, and stock cubes.

Meat and yeast extracts, pastes and pâtés made from fish and meat.

Be aware of hidden MSG. It is possible that any of the following may contain MSG:

Autolyzed yeasts, bouillon, barley malt, broth, calcium caseinate, flavourings (including those listed as natural), HVP (hydrolysed vegetable protein), HPP (hydrolysed plant protein), kombu extract, malt extract, seasonings, sodium caseinate, textured protein.

At the end of the five days, eat a meal that you would previously have eaten containing MSG and wait—an "immediate" reaction can take up to twelve hours to present itself.

Some people react immediately on eating any MSG whilst for others it is dose related—whereas one meal containing MSG may cause no problems, a second meal followed by a snack food with high levels can produce the symptoms. It is a cumulative process—you may be able to eat it once a week but not over a number of days in succession. If a large, for you, amount of MSG is ingested it is possible that the initial reaction will be severe but of short duration. You should not be fooled into thinking this is the only reaction you will get.

Monitor yourself carefully over the next few days and notice any additional changes such as bloating, rashes, mental confusion, false energy and headaches. If reactions have taken place you will be able to keep your MSG levels very low simply by avoiding it in its additive form. Some people's sensitivity is great enough to warrant that they also avoid foods that are very high in naturally occurring free glutamates.

Emsley and Fell list some of the foods with the highest amounts of naturally occurring MSG as follows (highest first):

Kelp, parmesan cheese, peas, tomatoes, corn, potatoes, spinach, chicken, carrots, beef, mackerel, pork, eggs.

Swain et al[71] list the following foods as being high in natural glutamate:

Vegetables: broccoli, mushroom, silver beet, English spinach, tomato, vegetable juice.
Fruit: grape, plum, prune, raisin, sultana.
Animal protein: processed meats.
Dairy: strong tasting cheese.
Condiments: miso, soy sauce, tempeh.

Don't forget that if you are attempting to lower your overall levels of MSG that you need to ensure that you are not taking in any of it in additive form (check the lists in the earlier part of this section).

If you had no reaction to added MSG but reacted to some of the foods in which it occurs naturally then you may have a problem with another food chemical such as salicylate rather than MSG.

Oxalic acid

Oxalic acid and oxalates are naturally occurring toxins in many foods. They are generally dealt with in the gastrointestinal tract and removed from the body in the faeces as calcium oxalate. In some people oxalates have been detected in the urine indicating that absorption from the gastrointestinal tract has taken place. It appears that this absorption takes place when calcium in food is tied up with other dietary components.

A build up oxalic acid can lead to kidney and bladder stones. Other symptoms that have been linked with high oxalic acid levels include abdominal pain, diarrhoea and sore throats. Plant leaves, especially rhubarb, beet tops and spinach, have the highest concentrations: the concentration is so high in rhubarb leaves that they have been classed as poisonous.

It is not possible to provide a full list of foods containing oxalic acid but the ones listed below have all been found to contain it.

> Beer, beetroot, blackberries, broad beans, celery, cocoa powder, gooseberries, green peppers, leeks, parsley, peanuts, pears, potatoes, red currants, runner beans, sorrel, spinach, strawberries, tea.

An average serving of each of these provides about 15mg of oxalate. Rhubarb has the highest amount, followed by spinach, beetroot, and cocoa powder. Star fruit[72] and high doses of ascorbic acid[73] have also been linked with oxalic acid problems. No oxalates have been identified in cereals, cheese, eggs, and most other fruit and vegetables.[74]

If you suspect an oxalic acid problem the general advice is to avoid the foods high in oxalate, limit your fat intake and increase your calcium intake. Do discuss these changes with your doctor first.

Phenylethylamine

See also *Amines*.

Phenylethylamine, derived from the amino acid phenylalnine, has been associated with changes in mood, behaviour and co-ordination. Emsley and Fell state that "there is no evidence that the body treats phenylethylamine as anything other than a chemical to be removed".[75] Cases of chocolate "allergy" have in fact turned out to be a problem with phenylethylamine. It appears that some people simply do not have sufficient quantities of the enzyme that breaks this amino acid down and prepares it for removal from the body.

Reactions to phenylethylamine have included:

Abdominal cramps, Diarrhoea, Dizziness, Flushing, Headache, Low blood pressure, Nausea, Respiratory problems, Urticaria.

The symptoms often appear to mimic an allergic reaction but when tested no allergy is identifiable. The phenylethylamine in chocolate could be one of the causes of chocolate related migraines.

Sandler et al identified a headache occurrence rate of 50% in those suffering from migraines when exposed to phenylethylamine as opposed to 6% of those receiving a placebo. It could be that some people are unable to fully metabolise phenylethylamine so leaving it in their systems longer and strengthening its effect on the vascular system.[76] Some migraine sufferers and children diagnosed with hyperactivity have been found to have elevated plasma phenylanine.[77]

Phenylethylamine is highly concentrated in high-protein foods such as meat and dairy products especially cheese. To reduce the level of the free form that is most likely to cause problems you would need to avoid all:

Processed meat and fish products, meat extracts, cheese, chocolate, wines and beer.

Products sweetened with aspartame.

To test for a problem with phenylethylamine avoid all the above foods, including aspartame, for at least two weeks and then reintroduce them gradually. Keep a food diary and remember that problems with phenylethylamine are probably dose related so a single test of, say, some processed meat is unlikely to provide a reaction unless you are extremely sensitive (do also remember that processed meats often contain other ingredients that can cause problems).

By carefully recording what you eat over a period of time, as well as any symptoms you experience, you should be able to see a pattern emerge that shows you how much food high in phenylethylamine you can tolerate before symptoms arise. If you use products containing aspartame please also read the section in *Sugars and Sweeteners*.

If there has been some improvement but symptoms, especially migraines, continue to persist then consider testing for a tyramine sensitivity—the foods that need to be avoided are very similar.

Purines

The production of uric acid is a normal bodily function. It is a waste product of digestion and is excreted via the kidneys as urine. In some individuals the removal of uric acid is impaired and it accumulates in the body eventually leading to unwanted symptoms.

Foods that contain the compound purine can raise the uric acid levels in the body leading, if you are susceptible, to conditions such as gouty arthritis or joint pain. These conditions are generally recognisable by their accompanying sudden and severe attacks of pain, redness and swelling of joints. The condition has been found to be helped by eating a low purine diet.

Gout generally comes on very suddenly with pain, swelling, warmth and redness usually in one joint. It has been commonly been associated with the big toe but can in fact afflict any joint. Some types of kidney stones can also be caused by uric acid build up and autism in some children has also been linked with an inability to correctly metabolise purines.[78]

Other problems have also been linked with purines. Moss reported on a study of the relationship between the consumption of alcohol, purines and boron, and the incidence of irritable bowel syndrome or frequent diarrhoea. The findings showed that individuals on diets high in alcohol, purines and boron had a higher prevalence of irritable bowel syndrome or frequent diarrhoea. The relationship was found to be significant.[79]

You will find it useful to test for purine sensitivity if:

- ◆ you have recurring gout like symptoms,

- ◆ only recently had a gout like episode but are also overweight and drink alcohol, or

- ◆ have irritable bowel syndrome that has not fully responded to other forms of dietary intervention.

It should be noted that not everyone with gout will have a purine sensitivity. As gout has become more prevalent there is now more awareness of the condition and many treatment protocols include some degree of dietary changes. If you have been given a diet to follow because of gout please do not stray from it without checking with your doctor first.

To test for a purine sensitivity, reduce the number of high purine foods in your diet for at least two weeks. Increase your intake of fruit and vegetables (choosing from those not on the lists) that you can eat as these increase the alkalinity of the blood and can help in the removal of excess uric acid. Avoid alcohol. High purine foods include[80]:

Meat especially red meat and offal, such as liver and kidneys, heart and sweetbreads.

Game, including pheasant, rabbit, and venison.

Seafood especially mussels, crab, shrimps and other shellfish, anchovies, herring, mackerel, sardines, sprats, whitebait trout, fish roe, caviar.

Yeast containing foods and beverages such as Marmite and beer.

Mushrooms and fungal proteins such as mycoprotein (Quorn), asparagus, cauliflower, spinach, lentils and soya beans.

For some the relief will be quite sudden but for others it can take time for the body to deal with removing the excess uric acid. If after a fortnight you are noticing some improvement you should maintain the diet. To actually test for a purine sensitivity is difficult as it is affected by the build up of uric acid to a level that is a problem for the individual—in some the response can be sudden, in others it can take weeks.

Persevere and monitor your success. As always with food testing, keep a food diary. It might be worth noting that strawberries, oranges, tomatoes and nuts, even though they are not high in purines, have triggered gout in some people.[81]

The other food that has increasingly been linked with gout is fructose.[82] Fructose rich drinks such as sugar sweetened soda and orange juice can increase serum uric acid levels and, hence, the risk of gout.[83] It is therefore probably best to also exclude these types of drinks. There will be a temptation to switch to sugar-free varieties but until you are sure that you need to eliminate the sugar drinks it would be best to stick to drinking water. Artificial sweeteners are often very complex products and adding them into your diet at this stage may lead to confusion with results of food testing.

Salicylates

The word "salicylate" is derived from the botanical name for the willow family "salicaceae" In 1838 salicylic acid was isolated from willow bark and, by 1899, acetylsalicylic acid was synthesised and marketed as aspirin. We come into contact with salicylate in two forms: In man-made substances such as medicines, solvents and perfume fixatives, and in its natural form in vegetables, fruit, spices, herbs and plants.

In nature, salicylates appear to exist as a natural preservative or insecticide protecting the plant and elongating its life span. The work of Anne Swain and others in Australia in the mid 1980s demonstrated the extent to which salicylate is present in food.[84] Virtually every meal we ever eat contains some salicylate and for most people this causes no problem but for an individual who is salicylate sensitive the consequences for their long-term health can be disastrous. The brain is often seriously affected as an overdose of salicylate first stimulates and then depresses the central nervous system leading to emotional and behavioural problems.

It has been particularly linked with hyperactivity as a result of the work of Dr Feingold in the 1970s. The results of research carried out by Williams et al support the theory that some food additives and industrial chemicals induce intolerance because of their aspirin-like properties.[85] A study of aspirin allergy by Speer et al found that 90% of those with aspirin sensitivity were also sensitive to inhalants, food or other drugs.[86] Others, including Thune and Granholt[87] have also found a cross-reactivity with aspirin. So, if you have an aspirin sensitivity consider testing salicylates more generally.

Many of the symptoms that arise as a result of salicylate intolerance mimic those of allergy but a reaction to salicylate is not an allergy. There is no simple method of testing to establish salicylate sensitivity—the most usual is the administration of an elimination diet followed by some form of challenge testing.

Salicylate is cumulative in the body and symptoms will only arise when the tolerance level of the individual has been exceeded. A large number of symptoms and conditions have been linked with salicylate and these are outlined below.

Mainly physical:
Abdominal pain, Aching legs, Asthma, Bed wetting, Bladder Problems, Dermatitis, Dizziness, Ear Infections, Eye muscle disorders, Fatigue, Headaches, Hives, Hypoglycaemia, Nasal polyps, Persistent cough, Physical sluggishness, Poor physical co-ordination, Psoriasis, Rhinitis, Sinusitis, Sleep disorders, Skin problems, Speech difficulties, Stomach irritation, Swelling of face, hands, feet, Tics, Tinnitus, Urticaria.

Emotions, Behaviour and Feelings
Accident proneness, Anxiety and agitation (no reason), Bouts of excessive energy followed by fatigue, Confused thinking, Depression, Distraction, Dyslexia, Excessive or constant talking, Hyperactivity, Impatience, Lack or loss of concentration, Memory problems, Mental sluggishness, Mood swings, Needing to be left alone, Nervousness, Poor self-image, Sudden bouts of paranoia, Sudden highs, Suicidal thoughts, Temper flare ups, Unpredictability, Workaholism

How do you know if you are salicylate sensitive?

Check the symptom list. How many of the symptoms do you currently have or have frequently had before? The greater the number the more likely you are to be sensitive. Have you had periods of times when you have experienced clusters of the symptoms? Salicylate sensitivity is generally a life-long condition and a pattern of symptoms and behaviour will be noticeable. Do spices, herbs or vegetables make you feel ill or do you have an aversion to them? This is not necessarily an indicator as we have often been conditioned about our responses but think back to childhood and how you responded to these at that time.

The only way to determine if you are salicylate sensitive is to reduce the level of salicylate in your system and the only way of doing this is to eat food containing no salicylate or very low levels. Once the body has eliminated the stored salicylate it is then possible to reintroduce foods containing a higher level and to assess the extent of any reaction.

If you suspect that salicylates may be a problem for you and you are taking any medication containing aspirin or another form of salicylate DO NOT undertake this test. Check ALL your medicines first and if in doubt ask your doctor. Ideally, all medications should also be additive (especially colour) free. If you are taking a salicylate medication then consult your doctor before even considering this test.

Please do take the above advice seriously. Aspirin, and other salicylate based drugs, contain a very concentrated form of salicylate. If you stop taking them, reduce the overall salicylate level in your system, and then take one you could be putting your life at risk. Death can result from anaphylactic shock.

As salicylate is cumulative in the body you need to lower your level over a period of at least two weeks. During this time you must be absolutely certain that you do not expose yourself to any high levels. Choose your fortnight with care as meals away from home will be very difficult to deal with. You can eat any amount of the foods listed as safe. If you are currently a vegetarian do not suddenly start eating meat, if you know that lettuce or one of the other foods makes you ill or you have an aversion to it then don't eat it—stick to foods you are used to eating, you can (if you want to) try the other ones later.

To make it easier for you the foods have been allocated a number so that you can keep score of how much salicylate you are eating—the score relates to an average portion. Your maximum allowance during this fortnight is FIVE a day and it is essential that you do not exceed this amount on any day. Keep a food diary and write down the total score for each day. Your food diary is going to become an incredibly important ally in unravelling your food sensitivities. Use it fully.

None of us are perfect and if you slip up don't beat yourself up about it. Correct it. If you find that on one day you unwittingly had a score of ten then make sure the next day's score is zero. Do not do the reverse—this means that if, for example, on the Friday, you scored three you must not increase Saturday's score to seven. KEEP TO FIVE. If you have slipped up on more than two consecutive days you will probably need to start your fortnight again.

At the end of the fortnight you will need to decide on the next stage. The degree of your sensitivity, your age, your overall health and the speed at which your body can detoxify will all have influenced what took place. You will probably find yourself in one of the following categories:

+ There was no noticeable change.

+ There was a gradual improvement in symptoms.

♦ There was no change at first then you had two or three days of feeling wonderful followed by days of being generally unwell and very tired—not too dissimilar to flu symptoms. Unless you have contracted a virus this is probably detoxification and nothing to be unduly concerned about.

♦ There was a substantial improvement in symptoms.

If you had no improvement in your symptoms then it is unlikely that you are salicylate sensitive. You can test this by eating as many foods from the high lists as you like. If after a fortnight these cause you no problem you can safely assume that you do not have a problem with salicylates. If there was a gradual improvement then you are probably salicylate sensitive. You can try to increase your salicylate level gradually. Increase your score allowance to ten a day over a two week period. If your symptoms begin to get worse again drop your level to five for a few days and then increase slowly until you find the level you can tolerate.

If you can tolerate a score of ten a day then increase to fifteen a day, once again for two weeks, and keep on doing this until you reach the level at which your symptoms reappear. The easiest way of dealing with a return of symptoms is drop your level to five for a few days and then take it back up when you feel better.

If you had a few days of feeling great and then feeling generally ill and tired it is likely that you have some degree of salicylate sensitivity. To give your body a chance to detoxify it is safest if you stay at this level for at least a further two weeks.

Testing for salicylate content in food has been slow in taking place. The lists that follow are based mainly on the research carried out by Swain et al.[88] Other studies have taken place but none has tested the same number of foods.[89,90] The findings from the other studies are explored in more detail in the *Salicylate Handbook.*[91]

The other issues about salicylate levels is that the amount may vary from different crops and harvests, not all foods have been examined, results have not been retested and, in the future, newer methods of analysis may be discovered. Having said that, the lists are more than adequate for establishing if you have a salicylate sensitivity and, if you do, will also enable you to establish your level of tolerance.

You are welcome to try foods not on the lists but so as not to confuse the results it would be advisable to treat them as suspect and only introduce them at a later stage when you can clearly determine what is happening. The categories of food are safe, very low, low, moderate, high, very high and extremely high.

If you get a reaction, be gentle with yourself. If salicylates affect your mind you may find it useful, when well, to write yourself a note you can read when a reaction takes hold—it should explain what is happening and reassure you that it will pass. If you have someone who understands what is happening talk to them—sometimes this helps minimise the effects of the anxiety.

Increase the number of safe fruit and vegetables you can eat as this increases the alkalinity of your blood. Taking extra Vitamin C can also help. If your blood sugar has been affected, don't worry. Eat lots of small meals for as long as you need—include "safe" treats. If you need to rest then take the time do so. It will pass. The length and severity of reactions will vary from individual to individual but, as it takes time for the body to eliminate salicylate, you can expect to experience symptoms for at least a few days.

Safe Salicylate Foods, Score = 0

Fruit: Banana, pear (peeled).

Vegetables: Bamboo shoot, cabbage (green/white), celery, dried green split peas, lentils, lettuce (iceberg), swede. Potatoes are fine but they must be of the old white variety and you must peel them.

Beans—dried (not borlotti). You may use canned beans but avoid any that have added ingredients such as sugar and salt.

Grains: Barley, buckwheat, millet, oats, rice, rye, wheat. To avoid additives and hidden preservatives, all bread, biscuits, cakes etc... should be home-made.

Seeds and nuts: Poppy seeds.

Sweeteners: Maple syrup, white sugar.

Meat, fish, poultry: Meat, fish, poultry and eggs are generally salicylate free but avoid liver and prawns and do not eat any processed meat.

Herbs, spices and condiments: Malt vinegar, saffron, sea salt, soy sauce.

Oils and fats: Cold pressed oils such as soy or sunflower. Butter. Margarine and processed rapeseed (canola), safflower, soya bean, sunflower oils although probably low in salicylate are likely to contain preservatives that may mimic salicylate reactions and are best avoided.

Dairy: Butter, cheese (not blue vein), milk, yoghurt—natural only but you can add your own fruit.

Misc: Carob powder, cocoa, tofu.

Beverages: Decaffeinated coffee, milk, ovaltine, home-made pear juice, soya milk, rice milk, water. Water should be the drink of your choice.

Very Low Salicylate Foods, Score=1

Fruit: Golden delicious apple without the peel (green variety only), paw paw, pomegranate, tamarillo.

Vegetables: Brussels sprouts, borlotti beans, chives, choko, garlic, green peas, leek, mung bean sprouts, red cabbage, shallot, yellow split peas.

Nuts and seeds: Cashew nuts.

Herbs, spices and condiments: Fennel—dried, fresh parsley.

Sweeteners: Golden syrup.

Meat and fish: Liver, prawns.

Low Salicylate Foods, Score = 2

Fruit: Fresh figs, lemon, mango, passion fruit, persimmon, red delicious apple (peeled), rhubarb.

Vegetables: Fresh asparagus, beetroot, cauliflower, green beans, onion, marrow, potato—with peel, pumpkin, tomato, turnip. Frozen spinach.

Seeds and nuts: Hazelnuts, pecan, sunflower seeds.

Herbs, spices and condiments: Fresh coriander leaves.

Oils and fat: Ghee.

Beverages: Dandelion coffee, shop bought pear juice.

Moderate Salicylate Foods, Score=3

Fruit: Custard apple, kiwi fruit, loquat, lychee, pear with peel.
Vegetables: Aubergine—peeled, carrot, lettuces other than iceberg, tomato juice, mushrooms. Tinned asparagus, beetroot, black olives, sweetcorn.
Seeds and nuts: Desiccated coconut, peanut butter, walnuts.
Sweeteners: Molasses.
Beverages: Coco-cola, rose hip tea.

High Salicylate Foods, Score=4

Fruit: Avocado, most other varieties of apples, cantaloupe melon, cherries, grapefruit, mandarin, mulberry, nectarine, peach, tangelo, watermelon.
Vegetables: Alfalfa sprouts, aubergine with peel, broad bean, broccoli, cucumber, tinned okra, parsnips, fresh spinach, sweet potato, tinned tomatoes and tomato puree, watercress.
Grains: Maize.
Seeds and nuts: Brazil nuts, macadamia nuts, pine nuts, pistachio, sesame seeds.
Herbs, spices and condiments: Yeast extracts.
Oils and fats: Almond oil, corn oil, peanut oil, sesame oil, walnut oil.
Beverages: Coffee.

Very High Salicylate Foods, Score=5

Fruit: Fresh apricots, blackberry, blackcurrant, blueberry, boysenberry, cranberry, fresh dates, grapes, guava, orange, pineapple, plum, strawberry, sultana.
Vegetables: Chicory, chilli peppers, courgette, endive, tinned green olives, peppers, radish, water chestnut.
Seeds and nuts: Almonds, peanuts with skins on.
Sweeteners: Honey.
Herbs, spices and condiments: Basil, bay leaf, caraway, chilli powder, nutmeg, vanilla essence, white pepper.
Oils and fats: Coconut oil, olive oil.
Beverages: Peppermint tea.

Extremely High Salicylate Foods, Score=6

Fruit: Dried apricots and dates. Currant, loganberry, prunes, raisin, raspberry, red currant.
Vegetables: Gherkins.
Herbs, spices and condiments: Allspice, aniseed, black pepper, cardamom, cayenne, celery powder, cinnamon, cloves, cumin, curry powder, dill, fenugreek, garam masala, ginger, liquorice, mace, mint, mustard, oregano, paprika, rosemary, sage, tarragon, turmeric, thyme, wine and cider vinegars.
Beverages: Cordials and fruit flavoured drinks, fruit and vegetable juices, tea.

Alcohol varies in amount. Given the difficulty in fully ascertaining the ingredients of alcoholic beverages, it is best to avoid drinking alcohol during the first two weeks. The following list can be only be treated as a very basic guide to levels. The safest course of action would be to introduce your favourite drink as a test.

Gin, whisky and vodka are probably safe.

Beer, brandy, cider, and sherry have a high salicylate content.

Liqueurs, port, rum, and wine are extremely high in salicylate.

Living with salicylate sensitivity is not easy. To maintain a level of salicylate that you can tolerate in your diet, you really are going to have to take responsibility for your diet—you can never allow anyone else to make a meal for you without first ensuring that they have a full list of the foods you can eat (it is easier to give a list of foods you can eat than those that need to be avoided).

Some food additives can also be a problem not necessarily because they contain any salicylate but because some of them mimic salicylate in the body. For example, adverse reactions to tartrazine are common in people who also react badly to salicylate,[92] probably because both are similar in structure and are detoxified in the same way. Similar problems have been found with the antioxidants BHA and BHT.[93]

Establishing a salicylate tolerance level is not an easy process and it can lead to a restrictive diet which is why many doctors advice against following one. Depending on your age and other factors unique to you, you may find that over a period of time you will be able to tolerate more salicylate. I suspect that at first, for some of us, our bodies are so relieved to have a reduction in the toxin that they rebel at the input of any but when the body has had time to recover it is more able to deal with eliminating salicylate and then accepts more.

Sadly, salicylates are found in a whole range of everyday products and, depending on your sensitivity, you will have to watch out for them. Perry et al have estimated that 12-20% of the salicylate in skin preparations is absorbed into the bloodstream via the skin.[94] As some ointments can contain high proportions of salicylate the risk for a sensitive person is serious. Ensure that none of the high and very high foods, especially herbs and spices, are present. Make sure you avoid anything with the word salicylate or salicylic within it. Some of the substances you need to watch out for include:

Acetylsalicylic acid, Almond oil, Aspirin, Benzoic acid, Benzoate—any form, Beta hydroxy, Birch, Bisabolol, Bismuth subsalicylate, Camphor, Castor oil, Homosalate, Hydroxybenzoate, Hydroxybenzoic, Menthol, Methyl salicylate, Methylene disalicylic acid, Oil of wintergreen, Ortho-hydroxybenzoic acid, Oxylsalicylate, Salicylaldehyde, Salicylanilide, Salicylic acid, Salicylic alcohol, Sodium salicylate, Stroncylate, Willow.

Carefully check medications, vitamins and other supplements, herbal remedies, cosmetics, creams and ointments, deodorants, toothpaste, teething gels, soap, shampoo, household cleaning products, air fresheners, insecticides, washing powders. Beware of perfumes as salicylate is often used as a fixative. It is best to avoid using perfume and scented products. Fragrance and colour free products are increasingly available.

I suspect that some people who tried a low salicylate diet for themselves or their children have run into this problem—an improvement followed later by seemingly salicylate unrelated problems. The symptoms are the same as before but you know the tolerance level has not been exceeded. If this happens check your environment—at work, home, school, wherever you spend time.

Crinon in an article on the health effects of airborne solvent exposure tell us that chemicals known as solvents are part of a broad class of chemicals called volatile organic compounds. These compounds are frequently used in a variety of settings and off-gas readily into the atmosphere. As a result of their overuse, they can be found in detectable levels in virtually all samples of both indoor and outdoor air. Once in the body they can lead to a variety of neurological, immunological, endocrinological, genitourinary, and hematopoietic problems.[95] Some individuals also have metabolic defects that diminish the liver's clearing capacity for these compounds.

Perfumes and solvents can give you these reactions and with these it is very difficult to know if they contain salicylate or not. The only way of knowing is to trust your nose which at first can lead to many unwanted reactions. If it all sounds difficult then you're reading the situation correctly. The positive side, and it is a massive one, is the better health that follows. Salicylate causes so many problems within the nervous system that all aspects of your life are affected by it—reducing the level substantially can, for someone with a salicylate sensitivity, lead to many positive changes.

Saponins

Saponins are a type of glycoside found in some plants. They are often particularly known for the soap-like foaming they produce when shaken in water.

Saponins occur in a wide variety of plant foods including soy and kidney beans and quinoa. Whilst some saponins are thought to have positive health benefits, they are also linked with adverse reactions in particular gastrointestinal reactions.

A large proportion of saponins can usually be removed by carefully washing the food in running water but some will inevitably remain in the food. There are many anecdotal reports of severe stomach cramping, vomiting and diarrhoea after eating foods like quinoa. We currently don't know if these problems have been caused by incorrect preparation/cooking or as a result of a sensitivity to either the food or the saponins.

A study by Fenwick and Oakenfull found the food plants, of the ones tested, that were highest in saponins to be

> Chickpeas, soya beans, lucerne (alfalfa) sprouts, navy beans, haricot beans, and kidney beans.

Tests showed that saponins were not destroyed by processing or cooking but that fermentation appears to make a difference—the saponin content of tempeh, a fermented soya bean product, was only half that of whole soya beans.[96]

If you suspect a problem with saponins then eliminate pulses and quinoa from your diet for seven days and monitor your progress when reinstating them into your diet—at this stage only add in ones that you ate before the test and please ensure that you follow preparation and cooking guidelines.

Serotonin

See also *Amines*.

The amine 5-hydroxytryptamine is what serotonin is known as in the world of science. Because of its actions as a neurotransmitter much has been written about the mood elevating qualities of serotonin but less has been written about the difficulties that an "excess" can cause for certain individuals.

Emsley and Fell cite the case of a fifty-two year old man who experienced one to two migraines a month and severe joint stiffness. After investigating his diet, which was high in meat, it was found that the cause of his problems was "a simple case of free amine overload due to a diet rich in tryptophan". Serotonin is produced from the amino acid tryptophan.[97]

The main symptom indicators would appear to be joint inflammation with no verifiable evidence of arthritis, and migraines not responding to other solutions. Other symptoms that have been noted include:

> Abdominal cramps, Breathing difficulties, Burning sensation in the mouth and throat, Dizziness, Flushing, Generalised itching, Headache, Nausea, Urticaria, Vomiting and diarrhoea.

Fish, meat, herbs and dairy products are all potentially high in tryptophan and a simple reduction in the amount if these eaten may be sufficient in establishing if there is a problem. It will also help to eat the freshest possible fish and meat, to avoid processed foods, sauces, and strong tasting cheeses.

Braverman lists the following foods as ones that contain tryptophan:

> Avocado, cheese, chicken, chocolate, cottage cheese, duck, egg, granola, luncheon meat, oat flakes, pork, sausage meat, turkey, wheat germ, whole milk, wild game, yoghurt.[98]

If you eat a lot of the same type of meat, fish or cheese you may want to consider varying the sources of your protein and adjusting how often you eat any particular food. Moderate amounts of serotonin have also been found in :

> Aubergine, black olives, broccoli, cantaloupe, cauliflower, dates, figs, grapefruit, honeydew melon, spinach.[99]

Keep a food diary and remember that problems with serotonin are probably dose related so a single test of one of the foods is unlikely to provide a reaction unless you are extremely sensitive. By carefully recording what you eat over a period of time, as well as any symptoms you experience, you should be able to see a pattern emerge that shows you how much food high in serotonin you can tolerate before symptoms arise.

Solanine

Solanine is a toxic alkaloid found in certain vegetables most notably potatoes. It probably acts as a preservative in the plants that works by making itself poisonous to fungi and bacteria and so preserving the life of the plant. It has been implicated in serious cases of food poisoning and has even resulted in death. A toxic dose will usually result in severe digestive upset and, possibly, trembling, weakness, breathing difficulties and paralysis.

McMillan et al reported on seventy eight schoolboys who became ill after eating potato at lunch, seventeen of them required admission to hospital. It was eventually found that the potatoes eaten by the boys who became ill were from an old batch and were found to be high in solanine. The symptoms were gastrointestinal, circulatory, neurological and dermatological with some boys being far more ill than others.[100]

Vegetables containing solanine are all members of the deadly nightshade family. Everybody should know that eating potatoes that are green is dangerous and should be avoided. Always ensure that your potatoes are thoroughly peeled with all the sprouting parts removed and if the potato is green—throw it away. Solanine is not destroyed by heating.

Aside from the rather serious toxic aspect of solanine there is a lesser problem of sensitivity that affects certain individuals. Ordinarily the liver will break down solanine and help us dispose of it but in some individuals this is not the case and an excess of solanine leads to inflammation.

If you have any condition involving painful joints you might like to try a solanine free diet for a while—improvements can be dramatic. Identified symptoms include:

Arthritis, Confusion, Drowsiness, Gastrointestinal problems, Hallucination, Migraine, Painful joints, Skin problems, Stomach irritation, Trembling.

Testing for a solanine problem is relatively straightforward as so few foods are involved. Simply eliminate them all from your diet for two weeks. If there is an improvement you will then have to decide on whether you wish to test or not. If there has been no change then solanine is not a problem for you.

Be cautious if you are still eating any processed food as potato starch creeps into products as diverse as soup, cakes and ice cream. The foods which contain solanine are:

Aubergine
Cayenne
Chilli
Green and red peppers
Paprika
Potato
Tomato

If you have experienced an improvement but feel you cannot live without some of these foods then gradually reintroduce them and increase the amount you eat. If you keep a careful note in your food diary you should be able to find the amount you can get away with before your problems return or the discomfort becomes unacceptable to you.

One way of reducing the solanine level is by removing the outer layer by peeling—this method can certainly be used with potatoes and, to a lesser extent, with tomatoes.

Sulphur and sulphites

"Sulphur" occurs naturally in a number of foods. "Sulphites" are sulphur based preservatives that are used to prevent or reduce discoloration of fruit and vegetables, prevent black spots on shrimp and lobster, inhibit the growth of micro-organisms in fermented foods such as wine, condition bread dough, and maintain the stability and potency of certain medications. Sulphites have been used since Roman times as preservatives in wine, sulphur dioxide was also used to sanitise wine and cider containers. Sulphites continue to be used in the wine making business in addition to their many other uses including the wet milling of corn to soften the kernel and facilitate the removal of corn starch.

A person can develop sulphite sensitivity at any point in life and no one knows, for definite, what triggers the sensitivity. Sulphites are broken down in the body by the same detoxification system that deals with other sources of sulphur in the diet such as amino acids like methionine and cysteine. In some individuals this detoxification system may not be working well and could give rise to a sulphite problem. Some countries have now prohibited the use of sulphites on fresh fruit and vegetables and insist on clear product labelling.

Sulphites have been most frequently linked with asthma. They are not generally seen as a cause of asthma but as a substance that can seriously exacerbate the condition. It has been estimated that between 5 and 10% of asthmatics are affected in this way. The Federation of American Societies for Experimental Biology (FASEB) in 1985 estimated that more than one million asthmatics are sensitive to or allergic to the substance.

Kochen in 1973 was among the first to suggest that the eating of sulphated food could cause bronchial problems. At the time he described the case of a child with mild asthma who repeatedly experienced shortness of breath, wheezing and coughing when exposed to dehydrated fruit that had been treated with sulphur dioxide.[101]

It became more accepted after work published by Baker et al,[102] and Stevenson and Simon,[103] both in 1981. Stevenson and Simon showed that challenges with potassium metabisulphite could produce significant changes in pulmonary function for some asthmatics. Other reported symptoms include flushing, tingling and faintness.

Problems with sulphites can result from ingestion, inhalation and topical application. Werth describes the case of an asthma sufferer who developed flushing, wheezing, and diaphoresis after inhaling vapours from a bag of dried apricots. In this case the person did not react to ingested sulphite when tested with a capsule of metabisulphite.[104]

Schwartz and Sher reported on a case in which breathing problems arose after an application of potassium metabisulphite solution to the eye during treatment for glaucoma.[105] Howland and Simon demonstrated that sulphated lettuce can trigger asthmatic reactions in asthmatics with a confirmed sulphite sensitivity.[106] Less serious reactions can include:

Abdominal pain and cramps, Chest tightness, Eczema, Headache, Hives, Itching, Localised angioedema, Minor breathing problems, Nausea and vomiting, Stomach ache, Throat irritation, Urticaria.

Changes in body temperature and heart rate have also been noted.[107] A typical low-grade reaction would be as follows:

after a meal you would suddenly find yourself a little tight chested and feeling as if you are starting with a cold. The sensation would probably disappear within a few hours and, most likely, you would forget about it. The symptoms need not all be physical.

Randolph cites cases in which individuals experienced mental symptoms including tension, nervousness, and depression. He says that "Sulfur can bring on acute mental and physical symptoms".[108] A sulphite sensitivity could also be a hidden problem for some individuals with irritable bowel syndrome as sulphites can interfere with the process of bacterial fermentation.

If you suspect a sulphite sensitivity and have breathing problems do NOT under any circumstances take this test without medical consent and supervision. Anaphylactic shock has been recorded as a result of sulphite reactions.

Foods high in naturally occurring sulphur have given rise to a number of symptoms including:

Abdominal pain, Bloating, Constipation, Diarrhoea, Dizziness, Generally feeling unwell, Headaches, Lack of co-ordination, Nausea and vomiting, Respiratory problems, Sneezing, Tight sensation in the chest. Tremors, Visual disturbances.

It is possible to be sensitive to naturally occurring sulphur and not to added sulphites and vice versa. It has also been found that sulphites destroy vitamin B1 which can be a problem for anyone on a poor diet. In some countries it is now banned from foods high in B1 such as meat. Eberlein-Konig et al also found that sulphites can contribute to UVB sensitivity.[109]

As sulphite is a product that is added to foods it is impossible to provide a full list of foods containing sulphite.

The following list, based in part on the re-examination of the GRAS status of sulfiting agents, is intended to serve only as a guideline—you must check labels of all foods for sulphite containing ingredients.[110]

Foods that are often very high in sulphites include:
Dried fruit, grape juice, lemon juice, lettuce, lime juice, molasses, sauerkraut juice, and wine.

Those that are often high in sulphites include:
Dried potato, fruit toppings, gravies, sauces, maraschino cherries, and wine vinegar.

Foods often with moderate amounts of sulphites include:
Corn starch, corn syrup, frozen potatoes, jams and jellies, maple syrup, mushrooms, pickles and relishes, sauerkraut, and shrimp.

Those often with low amounts of sulphites include:
Beer, coconut, dried cod, dry soup mixes, frozen pastries, gelatin, instant tea, malt vinegar, soft drinks, sugar, tinned potatoes,

Check all processed products including biscuits, crackers, enriched milk, meat and fish pies, pastes and ready meals, pies and pizza crusts, tortillas, any baked goods, any containing dried or processed fruit or vegetables, and all tinned foods. During the testing period avoid eating away from home especially in restaurants as in some countries sulphites are added to help keep food fresh.

These are the additives you need to watch out for:

E220 Sulphur dioxide
E221 Sodium sulphite
E222 Sodium hydrogen sulphite
E223 Sodium metabisulphite
E224 Potassium metabisulphite
E226 Calcium sulphite
E227 Calcium hydrogen sulphite
E228 Potassium hydrogen sulphite
E150(b) Caustic Sulphite Caramel
E150 Sulphite Ammonia Caramel

Unless you are extremely sensitive you will find that you can tolerate some sulphites. Your challenge will now to be find out just what you can get away with. Whilst establishing a safe level you would be advised to avoid take out, fast food and restaurant meals. Remember that exposure to sulphites can result from ingestion, inhalation and topical application.

If you have had any serious reactions in the past and you don't know what has caused them DO NOT undertake this test at home—discuss the way forward with your doctor. Whilst rare, anaphylaxis has been linked with sulphites so testing is safest under medical supervision.

Check all medicines, supplements, creams, toiletries, cosmetics and ointments as some of these can also contain sulphites. If any of these have been prescribed for you by a doctor you must not take this test—explain your concerns with your doctor and ask for their advice on how to establish if you have a sulphite problem whilst still being able to take the medication that you need.

At this point do not be too concerned about the foods that contain sulphur naturally—a complete elimination will probably be unnecessary and would cause you problems with eating sufficient protein.

Eliminate sulphites for at least ten days before testing. Follow the testing protocol given to you by your doctor or, if he was given you the go ahead to carry out the test at home, eat one of the foods you would have previously eaten that contained sulphites. If you have no reaction, gradually increase the number of foods with sulphites. If you experience any form of reaction—immediately stop the test and eliminate them from your diet once again.

If you found that you do have a sulphite sensitivity and have made some improvement but are still experiencing problems you may also need to reduce the amount of naturally occurring sulphur in your diet as well. Foods that contain natural sulphur include:

Bran, broccoli, Brussels sprouts, cabbage, cauliflower, cheese, dried beans, egg yolk, fish, garlic, lentils, meat, molasses, nuts, onions, pasta, wheat germ.

You need to take great care with this type of dietary restriction as you need to ensure that you are eating sufficient protein. If after two weeks you continue to experience problems then it is likely that you have a problem other than sulphur. Before embarking on further tests double and triple check the foods that you are eating, writing to manufacturers if need be, as residual sulphite concentrations can be found in many foods. Also ensure that you are avoiding corn products in case of sulphite contamination during rehydration processes.

Tannins

Tannins are naturally occurring chemicals found in a wide range of foods. It could be that, in a similar way to salicylates, they act as a form of natural protection for plants. They are also found in processed foods, medications and supplements where they are used as binders, coatings and preservatives.

The main symptom that has so far been linked with a tannin sensitivity is migraine.[111] So, if you suffer from migraines and no other test has worked, consider checking your tannin tolerance level.

As with most food chemicals, there is no definitive list of tannin levels in foods but the information in the lists below should help establish if tannins are a problem. The easiest way of testing for a tannin sensitivity is to remove all tannin foods, listed below, for two weeks and then gradually reintroduce them. You will need to keep a food diary to be able to closely monitor how you react and you should bear in mind that reactions may be delayed and may also be the result of a cumulative effect.

Legumes: The redder ones appear to have more than whiter beans but, for the test period, remove them all. It is worth noting that tannins tend to be more concentrated in the outer layers.[112]

Fruit: Berries such as blackberry, blueberry, cranberry, raspberry, strawberry.[113,114,115]

Nuts: Black walnut, cashew, English walnut, pecan, pistachio.[116]

Herbs and spices: It would appear that many herbs and spices contain tannins including cinnamon, cloves, cumin, tarragon, thyme, vanilla. As it is not currently possible to identify which are high and which are not, avoid all herbs and spices for the testing period.

Additives: You will need to avoid all added colours and flavourings as tannins can be used in the production of colours, flavour modifiers, and flavours such as butter, caramel, fruit, brandy, maple and nut.[117]

Cocoa: Cocoa powder and chocolate in all its forms.[118]

Misc: Any smoked foods.

Cheese: Avoid any cheese that has an added colour.

Beverages: Apple cider, beer, coffee, fruit juices, guarana, mate, tea, wine (especially red).[119]

If you have found yourself to be very tannin sensitive, you need to know that there are non-food products which may also give you a problem. Tannins are a sub-group of phenolics which are found in fragrances, paints, solvents, cleaning materials and the like.

Do not let this concern you at this stage. Continue with a low tannin diet and if you later get a re-occurrence of migraines then consider checking on the products commonly used, by yourself and others, in your home, work and social environment. This type of delayed reaction is not uncommon (often referred to as unmasking). Do not panic or necessarily suspect other foods. Keep a diary of all products used and how you feel in different places and you should soon be able to identify the primary culprits.

Tyramine

See also *Amines.*

Tyramine is produced from the amino acid tyrosine by enzymes produced by bacteria in both the gut and in food. In food, these bacteria increase in number, especially in ripe, fermented, some cooked, and badly stored food.

Tyramine, unlike some other amines, appears to serve no useful purpose in the body. Sadly, it is present in a large number of foods and in susceptible people can lead to high blood pressure, migraines, sleepiness and mood changes. It has been particularly linked with migraines because as a vasoactive amine it affects the blood vessels in a way which leads to changes in blood pressure and produces headaches.

Smith et al used double-blind placebo controlled challenges with forty five individuals with food induced migraine. Out of ninety four tyramine challenges, 80% resulted in a migraine.[120] Peatfield reports on a study of 577 people attending the Princess Margaret Migraine Clinic from 1989 to 1991 who were questioned about dietary triggers of their headaches. Of the 429 who had migraines, 16.5% reported that headaches could be precipitated by cheese or chocolate, and nearly always both.[121]

A sensitivity to alcohol, especially red wine and beer, was also found. They found that there was a definite statistical association between sensitivity to cheese/chocolate and to red wine and also to beer and concluded that cheese/chocolate and red wine sensitivity, in particular, have closely related mechanisms, in some way related more to migraine than to more chronic tension-type headache (no food sensitivities were reported in this category). They did not make the link between these food problems and tyramine but it seems likely to have been the cause.

Ghose and Turner found that women may become more sensitive to the effects of vasoactive amines such as phenylethylamine and tyramine in the perimenstrum.[122] So migraines at this point may be more likely to arise and could be misread as being caused by foods such as chocolate. The headache producing properties of tyramine are not restricted to individuals sensitive to an excess of it. Studies have shown that 100-125mg of tyramine leads to 90% of people experiencing a headache.

Tyramine sensitivity is an example of how easy it is to misread food intolerance—if your problem is tyramine and you test cheese (high in tyramine) in isolation then the migraines may abate. You will think the problem is the cheese and eliminate it from your diet. Your migraines may abate and then return leading to confusion because you thought you had identified the problem. At this point it is easy to get into a cycle of identifying and blaming other foods as well and limiting your diet unnecessarily because what has in fact happened is that your tyramine intolerance level has been exceeded. The problems caused by food chemicals has been grossly underestimated. They are difficult to ascertain because of their cumulative effect and the simple fact that we will all have different tolerance levels.

Tyramine can cause problems for people taking MAO (monoamine oxidase) inhibitors as monoamine oxidase in the gastrointestinal tract normally metabolises dietary monoamines such as tyramine. When this is blocked by drugs then more are absorbed into the body leading to symptoms such as palpitations, severe headaches and high blood pressure.

If you suffer from recurring migraines you may like to consider testing tyramine. Other implicating symptoms may also include:

High blood pressure, Palpitations, Agitation, Nervousness and Circulation problems.

The key factor in this test is to eat food as fresh as possible as the ageing, fermenting and ripening processes all increase the amount of tyramine.

To test for a tyramine sensitivity, avoid all tyramine foods listed below for at least seven days and then eat one of the foods from the list you most commonly eat but not cheese. If you immediately get a reaction then tyramine is a problem—stay of all tyramine foods for at least two weeks before trying again. On the second test try a different food from the list. Testing of cheese should only take place once you have established if you have a tyramine problem or not. The reason for this is a reaction to cheese could indicate a hidden milk intolerance problem rather than a problem with tyramine.

If on the first test there is no adverse reaction add a tyramine food each day. If you get no reactions over the next seven days then you are probably okay. If a reaction does occur then you are probably tyramine sensitive to some degree. In this case eliminate them all again and then gradually increase the number that you eat until you are able to gauge what amount you can tolerate. Full analysis of foods for tyramine has not been conducted but some information is available as it is a food chemical that must be avoided by anyone taking MAOI drugs if they are to avoid potentially serious reactions. There is no definitive list; the one below has been compiled from a number of sources including Joneja[123], Emsley and Fell,[124] and Diamond.[125] If your doctor has provided you with a list of foods to reduce or avoid then please stick with that list only.

Cheese: All cheese except for cottage cheese, cream cheese and ricotta cheese. Watch out for biscuits and snacks containing cheese.

Yeast: Brewer's yeast, sour dough, yeast extracts, yeast leavened breads made with fresh yeast (those made with baker's yeast are probably okay), yeast vitamin supplements, yeast found in processed foods.

Meat, poultry and fish: Avoid all game, liver pâtés, tinned, smoked, aged, pickled, fermented or marinated meat, fish and poultry products—this includes bacon, caviar, ham, hot dogs, leftovers, meat extracts, offal, pepperoni, salami and sausages. Buy fresh and eat within two days. Freshness is the key factor so be cautious in restaurants.

Fruit: Citrus fruit especially oranges, overripe bananas (also banana skins). You would be wise to avoid any overripe or spoiling fruit.

Vegetables: Aubergine, broad beans, green beans, bean pastes, fermented bean curds, fermented soya beans, mange tout, olives, pickles, sauerkraut

Condiments: Soy sauce, bean pastes, miso, teriyaki sauce.

Processed Food: Check the labels of any processed product to ensure avoidance of yeast and hydrolysed protein such as stock cubes, gravy, soup, sauces, stew mixes.

Beverages: Orange juice, tomato juice

Misc: Ginseng, tofu.

Alcohol: Beer including non-alcoholic brands. Wines including non-alcoholic brands. Whisky and liqueur.

MSG: It is probably also necessary to avoid all foods containing added MSG—check the section *MSG* for full details.

If you currently eat a lot of nut and/or seeds you might find it useful to also eliminate these from your diet during the testing period.

Tyramine has been identified in more than 200 foods. The foods with the highest amounts have been listed above. The following may require a limited intake—this will depend on the degree of your sensitivity:

Anchovies, avocados, beetroot, boiled eggs, buttermilk, caffeine, chocolate, colas, cream and cottage cheeses, cucumbers, curry powder, figs, fresh fish, lentils, mushrooms, pineapple, prunes, raisins, raspberries, raw onion red plums, salad dressings, sour cream, sourdough bread, spinach, sweet corn, tomato juice, yeast, yeast-leavened bread, vanilla extracts, yoghurt.

If you eat any of these try to eat them as fresh as possible. For the initial testing phase do not exclude them—just reducing your tyramine levels will probably be enough to provide an indication as to whether you have a problem with this amine or not. The fine-tuning can come later. This method will also prevent you from restricting your diet unnecessarily.

Other chemicals

This section contains a brief outline of some of the other chemicals found in food that can cause some people problems.

Aflatoxin

Aflatoxin is a mycotoxin produced by certain moulds. It can be found in foods as varied as nuts, peanuts, corn, milk, and dried fruit. Strict regulations govern the amount of permissible aflatoxin in foods, and poisoning in "developed" countries is rare.

Carvone

Carvone is a member of a family of chemicals called terpenoids. It is found naturally in many essential oils especially oil from seeds of caraway and dill. It is used in the production of flavours especially those that resemble spearmint, caraway, dill, mint and rye. It is also added to toiletries such as shampoos and hair conditioners.

One woman's head dermatitis was found to be caused by carvone.[126] Carvone has been responsible for cases of inflammation of the lips when it has been present in toothpaste.[127]

Glycyrrihizic Acid

Russo et al describe two cases of hypertension encephalopathy which resulted in pseudo hyperaldosteranism syndrome as a result of daily intake of low doses of liquorice. They propose that some people could be susceptible to low doses of glycyrrhizic acid because of a deficiency in a certain enzyme.[128]

Goitrogens

Goitre, thyroid enlargement, has been linked with over consumption of naturally occurring goitrogens in vegetables. The vegetables include Brussels sprouts, broccoli, cabbage, cauliflower, kale, mustard, radish, rapeseed, soya beans, and turnip. It appears that cooking reduces the goitre effect of these vegetables.

Hymenoptera insects

Red wine is often implicated in adverse reactions. The suspects have included sulphites, salicylates and histamine. Armentia introduced us to a new problem for some people by identifying allergic reactions, in some individuals, to Hymenoptera insects that fall into the wine when grapes are collected and pressed.[129]

Linamarin

Linamarin is found in cassava (manioc), an important vegetable in some parts of the world yet also inherently toxic. Linamarin can be converted to hydrocyanic acid and lead to toxic cyanide effects. Neurological disorders and thyroid enlargement have been found in people who eat large amounts of cassava that has not been adequately processed. To reduce toxic cyanide effects, cassava must be correctly processed by soaking, boiling, drying, and fermentation.

Moulds

Sometimes it is very difficult to identify the food culprit that is causing health problems. An example of this difficulty is when moulds are present in food either as a result of the way the food is processed or because of contamination.

Flavour-enhancing moulds are added to traditional foods such as dry sausage, salami, Spanish ham, and French cheese in Central and Southern Europe.[130]

In Northern Europe, the addition of moulds to meat products is not permitted but there are studies that have found contamination by Penicillium, Cladosporium, and Eurotium moulds in equipment and raw materials used during the manufacture of meat products. For example: In order to determine the mycobiota in processing areas of fermented sausage and liver pâté, filamentous fungi were isolated from air, equipment and raw materials in the processing areas of two fermented sausage processing plants and two liver pâté processing plants.

A total of three hundred and thirty six samples were examined. The diversity of filamentous fungi in the processing areas was high; at least seventeen different genera were identified. The main isolated genera were identified as Aspergillus, Botrytis, Cladosporium, Epicoccum, Eurotium, Penicillium, Phaeoacremonium and Phoma.

Of these, Penicillium and Eurotium were the most important for contamination of fermented sausage, whereas Penicillium and Cladosporium were most important for liver pâté. In total, sixteen Penicillium species were identified. Sorensen et al concluded that Penicillium species are the most important contaminants of the meat products because of their high prevalence in the production environment, their presence on meat products and their toxinogenic properties.[131]

Occupational respiratory diseases due to prolonged or repeated exposure to organic dust containing moulds (rhino conjunctivitis, asthma, hypersensitivity pneumonitis, and organic dust toxic syndrome) among food industry workers is well documented but food allergy to mould proteins is rare, with very few reports in the literature—two examples are given below.

Morriset et al presented two cases of recurrent angioedema after eating dry fermented sausages. These type of sausages are coated with various Penicillium strains and testing showed positive reactions in both cases to Penicillium.[132]

Bobolea et al presented the case of a twenty-four year old man diagnosed with rhino conjunctivitis and asthma due to allergy to pollens, mites, and moulds at the age of nine years. In the past year he had experienced two episodes of facial angioedema immediately upon eating a few slices of dry sausage, which he had previously tolerated. The symptoms subsided in less than six hours. He had avoided the sausage since then and tolerated all other types of meat products.

A range of tests were carried out. Skin prick tests were positive for grass pollen, house dust mites, and moulds (Alternaria alternata, Penicillium notatum, Mucor racemosus, and Pullularia, Stemphylium, Helminthosporum, and Fusarium spp.), and negative for all the food allergens tested. The prick-by-prick test was positive for the outer sausage skin and negative for the sausage meat.

The microbiologists isolated Penicillium and Mucor spp. in the sausage skin. A further test led to angioedema of the lips, tongue, and soft palate within five minutes. The diagnosis was facial angioedema after dry sausage ingestion due to IgE-mediated allergy to Penicillium and Mucor spp. The man was advised to avoid all products commonly contaminated with moulds such as dry fermented sausages, Spanish ham, foie gras, and French cheeses such as Roquefort and Camembert.[133]

If you eat fermented cheese or sausages and have problems you have been unable to link with a specific food it may be worth arranging for allergy tests to moulds.

Myristicin

Myristicin is found in nutmeg and carrots and can cause blurred vision, chest pressure, dry mouth, flushing, hallucinations, nausea, palpitations and a sense of impending doom. It is unlikely that you will be able to consume enough carrots to cause a problem but nutmeg poisoning has been reported.

Nickel

Flyvholm et al reviewed the nickel content of food as it is now thought that flare of hand eczema can occur after oral nickel exposure. The incidence of nickel allergy in the Danish population is thought to be 10% for women and 2% for men. Intake of nickel from the diet is estimated to be on average 150 micrograms per person per day.[134] Anderson et al found that nickel in tap water can also influence flare of hand eczema.[135] Nielsen et al found quite clear links between diet and flare of hand eczema due to nickel content.[136]

Vegetables and grains supply the average diet with nickel. Cocoa and chocolate, soya beans, oatmeal, nuts and legumes also have a very high nickel content. Consumption of these foods in large amounts can increase the nickel intake to 900 micrograms per person per day or more. It is possible for flare of hand eczema to take place within the range of 600-5,000 micrograms. It would be necessary to establish the individual threshold.

Nickel content does vary. Joneja's review of nickel levels in common foods has the highest as being buckwheat, oats, dark chocolate, peanuts, walnuts, flaxseed, cocoa powder, tea, and legumes.[137]

Avoiding canned and processed foods would seem to be helpful as Smart and Sherlock found high concentrations in canned vegetables, sugars and preserves (also in bread and cereals) and suggest that nickel content can increase as a result of food processing.[138]

Nitrates

Nitrates and nitrites have been used for centuries to preserve meat. The problem with them occurs when nitrate combines with certain other compounds in the digestive system it forms nitrosamines which are thought to be powerful cancer causing chemicals. There have been studies that have linked the regular ingestion of nitrates with some forms of cancers especially in the intestines.[139]

Nitrates have also been linked with less serious forms of sensitivity. For example, a case of severe itching was found to be caused by nitrates—a forty-year old woman experienced severe itching on the arms and back. Testing after an elimination diet established that nitrates were the cause; within three hours of ingesting sodium nitrate the itching emerged and remained for four days, nitrate intolerance was diagnosed.[140]

Many processed and cured meats contains added nitrates. The additives to avoid are:

E249 Potassium nitrite
E250 Sodium nitrite
E251 Sodium nitrate
E252 Potassium nitrate

Phenols

Phenolic compounds are found in a wide range of foods. These are natural substances that colour and flavour foods. The fact that they are toxic could be nature's way of protecting itself against micro-organisms and aiding the dispersal, and germination, of the seeds. Generally our body eliminates these toxins with no difficulty but for some people they cause problems. The discovery of phenolic compounds led Dr Robert Garner to devise a neutralisation technique using dilutions of these substances to stop his own allergic reactions. Some examples of phenols are:

Eugenol found in almond, beef, carrot, celery, cheese, milk, orange, pea, soya bean, tomato.

Piperine found in beef, beet sugar, cheese, chicken, cow's milk, grape, lamb, onion, pea, potato, soya bean, tomato, yeast.

Cinnamic acid is one of the better known ones, its precursor in most plants is phenylalanine. Cinnamic acid gets its name from oil of cinnamon where it was first discovered. Its presence may reach as much as 13 mg/100g in such foods as apples or 14 mg/100g in sweet cherries and 14.5 mg/100g in grapes (68).[141]

The amount and concentration of phenols varies greatly from plant to plant. How they affect health is complex as it is influenced by their interaction with each other and with other chemical compounds. As yet it is not clearly known which phenols are beneficial, which are harmful and which may lead to sensitivities.

Propionates

The food additive "calcium propionate" has been linked with some migraine headaches and skin rashes.

A report in 2002 also linked it with behaviour problems (irritability, restlessness, inattention, and sleep disturbance) in children.[142]

The propionates, listed below, are quite frequently found in bread and other products made with flour.

E281 Sodium Propionate
E282 Calcium Propionate
E282 Potassium Propionate

Tin

Tin plate is commonly used in the construction of metal cans for foods. If the tins are not adequately lined when used for acidic foods such as tomato juice and fruit cocktail then tin intoxication can take place. Tin is poorly absorbed and hence the early symptoms are bloating, nausea, abdominal cramps, vomiting, diarrhoea and headache within thirty minutes to two hours.[143]

References

[1] Emsley J, Fell P. Was it something you ate? Food Intolerance: what causes it and how to avoid it. O.U.P. 1999.

[2] Joneja JV. Dietary Management of Food Allergies and Intolerances: A Comprehensive Guide. Second edition. J.A. Hall Publications, 1998.

[3] Emsley J, Fell P. Was it something you ate? Food Intolerance: what causes it and how to avoid it. O.U.P. 1999.

[4] Jacobson DW. Adverse reactions to benzoates and parabens. In: Metcalfe DD, Sampson HA, Simon RA. (eds) Food Allergy: Adverse reactions to foods and food additives, 2nd ed. Blackwell Science 1997, 375-386.

[5] Wuthrich B, Fabro L. Acetylsalicylic acid and food additive intolerance in urticaria, bronchial asthma and rhinopathy. Schweiz Med Wochenschar 1981;111(39):1445-50.

[6] Juhlin L, Michaelsson G, Zetterstrom O. Urticaria and asthma induced by food-and-drug additives in patients with aspirin hypersensitivity. J Allergy Clin Immunol 1972;50:92-98.

[7] Michaelsson G, Juhlin L. Urticaria induced by preservatives and dye additives in foods and drugs. Br J Dermatol 1973;88:525-32.

[8] August PJ. Successful treatment of urticaria due to food additives with sodium cromoglycate and exclusion diet. In: Pepys J, Edward AM (eds). The Mast Cell: its role in health and disease. Pitman Medical 1979;584-590.

[9] Gibson A, Clancy R. Management of chronic idiopathic urticaria by the identification and exclusion of dietary factors. Clin Allergy 1980;10:699-704.

[10] Ortoloni C, Pastorello E, Luraghi MT, Della Torre F, Bellani M, Zanussi C. Diagnosis of intolerance to food additives. Ann Allergy 1984;53:587-91.

[11] Chafee RH, Settipane GA. Asthma caused by FD&C approved dyes. J Allergy 1967;40:65-72.

[12] Asero R. Sodium benzoate-induced pruritus. Allergy. 2006 Oct;61(10):1240-1.

[13] Joneja JV. Dietary Management of Food Allergies and Intolerances: A Comprehensive Guide. Second edition. J.A. Hall Publications, 1998.

[14] Bolton S, Feldman M, Null G, Revici E, Stumper L. A pilot study of some physiological and psychological effects of caffeine. J Orthomolecular Psych 1985;13(1).

[15] Bolton S, Null G. Caffeine: Psychological Effects, Use and Abuse; Orthomolecular Psych 1981;10(2):202-211.

[16] Spiller GA. The methylxanthine beverages and foods: chemistry, consumption and health effects. Prog Clin Biol Res 1984;1: 854-6.

[17] Marchbanks CR. Drug-drug interactions with fluoroquinolines. Pharacotherapy 1993,13(pt2):23S-28S.

[18] Silverman K, Evans SM, Strain EC, Griffiths RR. Withdrawal syndrome after the double-blind cessation of caffeine consumption. New Eng J Med 1992;327:1109-14.

[19] Charney DS, Heninger GR, Jatlow PI. Increased anxiogenic effects of caffeine in panic disorders. Arch Gen psychiatry 1985;42:233-43.

[20] Davis RE, Osorio I. Childhood caffeine tic syndrome. Pediatrics 1998;101(6):E4.

[21] Greden JF. Anxiety or caffeinism - a diagnostic dilemma. Am J Psychiatry 1974;131:1089-92.

[22] Gancedo SQ, Freire P, Rivas MF, Davila I, Losada E. Urticaria from caffeine. J Allergy Clin Immunol 1991;88:680-81.

[23] Pola J, Subiza J, Armentia A, Zapata C, Hinjosa M, Losada E, Valdivieso R. Urticaria caused by caffeine. Ann Allergy 1988;60:207-8.

[24] Fernández-Nieto M, Sastre J, Quirce S. Urticaria caused by cola drink. Allergy. 2002 Oct;57(10):967-8.

[25] MAFF Survey of caffeine and other methylxanthines in energy drinks and other caffeine-containing products (updated). Food Surveillance Information Sheet, (144): 26pp, March 1998 (No 103 revised).

[26] http://www.mayoclinic.com/health/caffeine/AN01211

[27] Rozin P, Leveine E, Stoess C. Chocolate craving and liking. Appetite 1991;17:199-212.

[28] Serio FG, Siegal MA, Slade BE. Plasma cell gingivitis of unusual origin: A case report. J Periodontol 1991;62:390-3.

[29] Myers BM, Smith L, Graham DY. Effect of red pepper and black pepper on the stomach. Am J Gastronterol 1987;82:211-14.

[30] Atherton DJ. Diagnosis and management of skin disorders caused by food allergy. Ann Allergy 1984;53(6Pt2):623-8.

[31] Feighery C. Coeliac Disease. BMJ 1999;319:236-39.

[32] Braly J., Hoggan R. Dangerous Grains. Avery, 2002.

[33] Wray D. Gluten-sensitive recurrent aphthous stomatitis. Dig Dis Sci 1981;26:737-740.

[34] Philpott W H, Kalita D H. Brain Allergies: The Psychonutrient and Magnetic Connections. Keats 2000.

[35] Braly J., Hoggan R. Dangerous Grains. Avery, 2002.

[36] Janatuinen E K, Kemppainen T A, Pikkarainen P H, Holm K H, Kosma V-M, Uusitupa M I J, Maki M, Julkunen R J K. Lack of cellular and humoral immunological responses to oats in adults with coeliac disease. Gut 2000;46:327-31.

[37] Hallert C, Olsson M, Storsrud S, Lenner RA, Kilander A, Stenhammar L. Oats can be included in gluten-free diet. Lakartidningen 1999;96(30-31):3339-40.

[38] Reunala T, Collin P, Holm K, Pikkarainen P, Miettinen A, Vuolteenaho N, Maki M. Tolerance to oats in dermatitis herpetiformis. Gut 1998;43(4):490-3.

[39] Gottschall E. Whatever happened to the cure for coeliac disease? Nutritional Therapy Today. 1997:7(1):8-11.

[40] Faulkner-Hogg KB, Selby WS, Loblay RH, Morrow AW. . Dietary analysis in symptomatic patients with coeliac disease on a gluten-free diet: the role of trace amounts of gluten and non-gluten food intolerances. Scand J Gastroenterol 1999;34(8):784-9.

[41] Braly J., Hoggan R. Dangerous Grains. Avery, 2002.

[42] Faulkner-Hogg KB, Selby WS, Loblay RH, Morrow AW. . Dietary analysis in symptomatic patients with coeliac disease on a gluten-free diet: the role of trace amounts of gluten and non-gluten food intolerances. Scand J Gastroenterol 1999;34(8):784-9.

[43] FSA. Claims about gluten: consumer advice. Jan. 2012. http://www.food.gov.uk/multimedia/pdfs/publication/glutenconsumer.pdf

[44] Braly J., Hoggan R. Dangerous Grains. Avery, 2002.

[45] Emsley J, Fell P. Was it something you ate? Food Intolerance: what causes it and how to avoid it. O.U.P. 1999.

[46] Ibid.

[47] Maintz L, Novak N. Histamine and histamine intolerance. Am J Clin Nutr. 2007 May;85(5):1185-96.

[48] Wantke F, Gotz M, Jarisch R. The histamine-free diet. Hautarzt 1993;44(8):512-6.

[49] Doeglas HMG, Huisman J, Nater J P. Histamine intoxication after cheese. Lancet 2;1967:1361-2.

[50] Motil KJ, Scrimshaw NS. The role of histamine in scombroid poisoning. Toxicity Lett 1979;2:219.

[51] Morrow JD, Margolies GR, Rowland BS, Roberts LJ. Evidence that histamine is the causative toxin of scombroid-fish poisoning. N Eng J Med 1991; 324:716-20.

[52] Joneja JV. Dietary Management of Food Allergies and Intolerances: A Comprehensive Guide. Second edition. J.A. Hall Publications, 1998.

[53] Maintz L, Novak N. Histamine and histamine intolerance. Am J Clin Nutr. 2007 May;85(5):1185-96.

[54] American Academy of Allergy and Immunology Committee on Adverse Reactions to Foods. US Dep H&HS, NIH Publications; 1984:84-2442.

[55] Baldwin JL. Pharmacologic food reactions. In: Metcalfe DD, Sampson HA, Simon RA. Food Allergy: Adverse reactions to foods and food additives, 2nd ed. Blackwell Science 1997, 419-29.

[56] Maintz L, Novak N. Histamine and histamine intolerance. Am J Clin Nutr. 2007 May;85(5):1185-96.

[57] Gilbert RJ. Healthy eating day. Communicable Disease Report 1988;33:3-4.

[58] Emsley J, Fell P. Was it something you ate? Food Intolerance: what causes it and how to avoid it. O.U.P. 1999.

[59] D'Adamo PJ. Eat Right 4 Your Type: The Individualized Diet Solution to Staying Healthy, Living Longer & Achieving Your Ideal Weight. 1997 G. P. Putnam's Sons.

[60] Freed D L J. Do dietary lectins cause disease? BMJ 1999;318:1023-24.

[61] Hamid R, Masood A. Dietary Lectins as Disease Causing Toxicants. Pakistan Journal of Nutrition 8 (3): 293-303, 2009.

[62] Ramona L. Rea, Lilian U. Thompson, David J.A. Jenkins, Lectins in foods and their relation to starch digestibility, Nutrition Research, Vol 5: 9, 1985, 919-929.

[63] Cordain L. Cereal grains: humanity's double-edged sword. World Rev Nutr Diet. 1999;84:19-73.

[64] Allen DH, Baker GJ. Chinese restaurant asthma. N Eng J Med 1981;278:796.

[65] Allen DH, Delohery J, Baker G. Monosodium L-glutamate-induced asthma. J Allergy Clin Immunol 1987;80(4):530-7.

[66] Blaylock RL. Excitotoxins: The Taste that Kills. Health Press, 1997.

[67] Squire EN. Angioedema and MSG. Lancet 1987;24:167-72.

[68] Botey J, Cozzo M, Marin A, Eseverri JL. Monosodium glutamate and skin pathology in pediatric allergology. Allergol Immunopathol (Madr). 1988 Nov-Dec;16(6):425-8.

[69] Blaylock RL. Excitotoxins: The Taste that Kills. Health Press, 1997.

[70] Joneja JV. Dietary Management of Food Allergies and Intolerances: A Comprehensive Guide. Second edition. J.A. Hall Publications, 1998

[71] Swain AR, Soutter VL, Loblay RH. Friendly Food: The essential guide to avoiding allergies, additives and problem chemicals. Murdoch Books, 2004.

[72] Fang,H.-C., Lee,P.-T., Lu,P.-J., Chen,C.-L., Chang,T.-Y., Hsu,C.Y., et al. Mechanisms of star fruit-indused acute renal failure. Food and Chemical Toxicology. 2008; 46: 1744-52.

[73] Barness, L.A. Safety considerations with high ascorbic acid dosage. Annals of the New York academy of science. 1975; 258: 523-8.

[74] Emsley J, Fell P. Was it something you ate? Food Intolerance: what causes it and how to avoid it. O.U.P. 1999.

[75] Emsley J, Fell P. Was it something you ate? Food Intolerance: what causes it and how to avoid it. O.U.P. 1999.

[76] Sandler M, Youdin MBH, Hannington E. A phenylethylamine oxidising defect in migraine. Nature 1974;350:335-7.

[77] Braverman ER. The Healing Nutrients Within. Keats 1987.

[78] http://purineresearchsociety.org/

[79] Moss M. Purines, Alcohol and Boron in the Diets of People with Chronic Digestive Problems. J Nutrit Env Med 11(1):23-32.

[80] Jordan KM, Cameron JS, Snaith M, Zhang W, Doherty M, et al. (SGAWG). British Society for Rheumatology and British Health Professionals in Rheumatology guideline for the management of gout. Rheumatology (Oxford). 2007 Aug;46(8):1372-4.

[81] UK Gout Society. All about gout and diet. http://www.ukgoutsociety.org/docs/2009FinalDietsheet.pdf

[82] Zychowicz ME. Gout: no longer the disease of kings. Orthop Nurs. 2011 Sep-Oct;30(5):322-30; quiz 331-2.

[83] Choi HK, Willett W, Curhan G. Fructose-rich beverages and risk of gout in women. JAMA. 2010 Nov 24;304(20):2270-8.

[84] Swain A , Dutten SP, Truswell AS. Salicylates in Food. J Am Dietetic Assoc 1985;85(8).

[85] Williams WR et al. Aspirin-like effects of selected food additives and industrial sensitising agents. Clin Exp Allergy 1989;19(5):533-37.

[86] Speer F et al. Aspirin allergy. Ann Allergy 1981 46(3):123-6.

[87] Thune P, Granholt A. Provocation tests with antiphologistica and food additives in recurrent urticaria. Dermatogica 1975;151:360-64.

[88] Swain A , Dutten SP, Truswell AS. Salicylates in Food. J Am Dietetic Assoc 1985;85(8).

[89] Wood A, Baxter G, Thies F, Kyle J, Duthie G. A systematic review of salicylates in foods: estimated daily intake of a Scottish population. Mol Nutr Food Res. 2011 May;55 Suppl 1:S7-S14.

[90] Scotter MJ, Roberts DPT., Wilson LA, Howard FAC, Davis J, Mansell N. Free salicylic acid and acetyl salicylic acid content of foods using gas chromatography–mass spectrometry. Food Chemistry, Vol 105, 1, 2007, 273-279 .

[91] Race, S. The Salicylate Handbook. Tigmor Books, 2012.

[92] Settipane GA, Pudupakkam RK. Aspirin intolerance III: sub-types, familial occurrence and cross reactivity with tartrazine. J Allergy Clin Immunol 1975;56:215-21.

[93] Fisherman EW, Cohen GN. Aspirin and other crossreacting small chemicals in known aspirin intolerant patients. Ann Allergy 1973;31:476-84.

[94] Perry CA et al. Health effects of salicylates in foods and drugs. Nutrition reviews 1996;54(8):225-240.

[95] Crinnion W J. Environmental Medicine, Part 2 - Health Effects of and Protection from Ubiquitous Airborne Solvent Exposure. Altern Med Rev 2000;5(2):133-143.

[96] Fenwick DE, Oakenfull D. Saponin content of food plants and some prepared foods. J Sci Food Agric. 1983 Feb;34(2):186-91.

[97] Emsley J, Fell P. Was it something you ate? Food Intolerance: what causes it and how to avoid it. O.U.P. 1999.

[98] Braverman ER. The Healing Nutrients Within. Keats 1987

[99] Feldman JM, Lee EM. Serotonin content of foods: effect on urinary excretion of 5-hydroxyindoleacetic acid. Am J Clin Nutr 1985;42:639-43.

[100] McMillan M, Thompson JC. An outbreak of suspected solanine poisoning in schoolboys: Examinations of criteria of solanine poisoning. Q J Med 1979;48(190):227-43.

[101] Kochen J. Sulfur dioxide, a respiratory tract irritant, even if ingested. Letter. Pediatrics 1973;52:145-6.

[102] Baker GJ, Collet P, Allen DH. Bronchospasm induced by metabisulfite-containing foods and drugs. Med J Aust 1981;2:614-16.

[103] Stevenson DD, Simon RA. Sensitivity to ingested metabisulfites in asthmatic subjects. J Allergy Clin Immunol 1981;68:26-32.

[104] Werth GR. Inhaled metabisulfite sensitivity. Letter. J Allergy Clin Immunol 1982;70:143.

[105] Schwartz H, Sher TH. Bisulfite intolerance manifest as bronchospasm following topical dipirefrin hydrochloride therapy for glaucoma. Letter. Arch opthalmol 1985;103:14-15.

[106] Howland WA, Simon RA. Restaurant-provoked asthma: sulfite sensitivity? J Allergy Clin Immunol 1985;75:145.

[107] Tollefson L. Quarterly report on consumer complaints on sulfiting agents. US Dept H&H Services, memo, April 2 1986:1-7.

[108] Randolph TG, Moss R W. An Alternative Approach to Allergies: The new field of clinical ecology unravels the environmental causes of

mental and physical ills (revised edition). Perennial Library, Harper & Row 1990.

[109] Eberlein-Konig B, Bergner T, Diemer S, Przybilla B. Evaluation of phototoxic properties of some food additives: sulfites exhibit prominent phototoxicity. Acta Derm Venereol 1993;73(5):362-4.

[110] LSRO (Life science research office). The re-examination of the GRAS status of sulfiting agents. Fed Am Socs for Exp Biology, Jan 1985.

[111] Mather M. Migraines and tannins-any relationship? Headache 1997;37(8):529.

[112] Gupta YP. Anti-nutritional and toxic factors in food legumes: a review. Plant Foods Hum Nutr. 1987;37(3):201-28.

[113] Vattem DA, Ghaedian R, Shetty K (2005). "Enhancing health benefits of berries through phenolic antioxidant enrichment: focus on cranberry". Asia Pac J Clin Nutr 14 (2): 120–30.

[114] Puupponen-Pimiä R, Nohynek L, Meier C, et al. (April 2001). "Antimicrobial properties of phenolic compounds from berries". J. Appl. Microbiol. 90 (4): 494–507

[115] http://clients.teksavvy.com/~mmather/foods.html

[116] http://www.widomaker.com/~jnavia/tannins/tannlist.htm

[117] http://www.allallergy.net/fapaidfind.cfm?cdeoc=1977

[118] Natsume M., Osakabe N., Yamagishi M., Takizawa T., Nakamura T., et al. Analyses of polyphenols in cacao liquor, cocoa, and chocolate by normal-phase and reversed-phase HPLC. Bioscience, Biotechnology and Biochemistry 64:2581-2587.

[119] http://clients.teksavvy.com/~mmather/foods.html

[120] Smith I, Kellow AH, Hannington E. A clinical and biochemical correlation between tyramine and migraine headache. Headache 1970;10:43-51.

[121] Peatfield RC. Relationships between food, wine, and beer-precipitated migrainous headaches. Headache 1995;35(6):355-7.

[122] Peatfield RC. Relationships between food, wine, and beer-precipitated migrainous headaches. Headache 1995;35(6):355-7.

[123] Joneja JV. Dietary Management of Food Allergies and Intolerances: A Comprehensive Guide. Second edition. J.A. Hall Publications, 1998.

[124] Emsley J, Fell P. Was it something you ate? Food Intolerance: what causes it and how to avoid it. O.U.P. 1999.

[125] Diamond, S. Conquering Migraine. Fireside, 2001.

[126] Quertermous J, Fowler JF Jr. Allergic contact dermatitis from carvone in hair conditioners. Dermatitis. 2010 Apr;21(2):116-7.

[127] Corazza M, Levratti A, Virgili A. Allergic contact cheilitis due to carvone in toothpastes. Contact Dermatitis. 2002 Jun;46(6):366-7.

[128] Russo S, Mastropasqua M, Mosetti MA, Persegani C, Paggi A. Low doses of liquorice can induce hypertension encephalopathy. Am J Nephrol 2000, 20(2):145-8.

[129] Armentia A. Adverse reactions to wine: think outside the bottle. Curr Opin Allergy Clin Immunol. 2008 Jun;8(3):266-9.

[130] López-Díaz TM, Santos JA, García- López ML, Otero A. Surface mycoflora of a Spanish fermented meat sausage and toxigenity of Penicillium isolates. Int J Food Microbiol. 2001;68:69-74.

[131] Sorensen LM, Jacobsen T, Nielsen PV, Koch AG. Mycobiota in the processing areas of two different meat products. Int J Food Microbiol. 2008;124:58-64.

[132] Morisset M, Parisot L, Kanny G, Moneret-Vautrin DA. Food allergy to moulds: two cases observed after dry fermented sausage ingestion. Allergy. 2003;58:1203-4.

[133] I Bobolea, P Barranco, J Jurado-Palomo, M Pedrosa, S Quirce. Allergy to Dry Fermented Sausage. J Investig Allergol Clin Immunol 2009; Vol. 19(4): 324-335.

[134] Flyvholm MA, Nielsen GD, Andersen A. Nickel content of food and estimation of dietary intake Z Lebensm Unters Forsch 1984;179:427-31.

[135] Anderson KE, Nielsen GD, Flyvholm MA, Fregert S, Gruvberg B. Nickel in tap water. Contact dermatitis. 1983;9(2):140-3.

[136] Nielsen GD, Jepsen LV, Jorgensen PJ, Grandjean P, Bradnrup Y. Nickel-sensitive patients with vesicular hand eczema: oral challenge with a diet naturally high in nickel. Br J Dermatol 1990;122(3) 299-308.

[137] Joneja JV. Dietary Management of Food Allergies and Intolerances: A Comprehensive Guide. Second edition. J.A. Hall Publications, 1998.

[138] Smart GA, Sherlock JC. Nickel in foods and the diet. Food Addit Contam 1987;4(1):61-71.

[139] Ferrucci LM, Sinha R, Huang WY, Berndt SI, Katki HA, Schoen RE, Hayes RB, Cross AJ. Meat consumption and the risk of incident distal colon and rectal adenoma. Br J Cancer. 2011 Dec 13.

[140] Asero R. Nitrate intolerance. Allergy 2000;55:678–679.

[141] Charambous I, ed. The Quality of Foods And Beverages, Vol. 1. Academic Press, 1981.

[142] Dengate S, Ruben A. Controlled trial of cumulative behavioural effects of a common bread preservative. J Paediatr Child Health 2002;38(4):373-6.

[143] Barker WH Jr, Runte V. Tomato juice associated gastroenteritis, Washington and Oregon, 1969. Am J Epidemiol 1972;96:219-26.

5 Individual Foods

Testing of individual foods does contain an element of risk which is why I advice that you carry out these tests in conjunction with your doctor. Even if you have been given the go-ahead to test a food at home I would advise that somebody is with you for at least the first two to three hours after testing—if you have a severe reaction they can obtain medical help for you. Remember, anaphylaxis can be life threatening.

The other advantage of having someone present is that we are not always very good at noticing changes within ourselves. Although you will know if you have a headache, rash or stomach ache easily enough, a change in how you are speaking or behaving is not always easy to detect. These behaviour changes are difficult to spot because if you have been reacting in the same way to a particular food for many years the change may not seem unusual to you, in fact it may feel familiar and "safe".

If you already avoid a food then do not test it. You are probably avoiding it for a very good reason. This of course does not apply to foods that you have never tried.

It is impossible to provide a full list of potential symptoms for each food as any food can cause any problem—it is very much an individual specific response. In some cases it has been possible to draw up a list of the type of symptoms that have been reported but these lists are only telling us some of the recorded symptoms. Please remember that:

Any food can cause any symptom.

When testing a food eat it in its most simple form. For example, testing milk by eating ice cream is not okay, nor is testing hazelnuts by eating a chocolate bar containing them. Keep it simple. In the examples given above simply drink some milk or eat some hazelnuts on their own. If at all possible use organic foods for testing—this is to avoid conflicting results due to pesticides. If you cannot find an organic version do still carry out the test and if you are uncertain of the results simply repeat the test.

Chocolate

Chocolate is commonly seen as an allergenic food but very few actual "allergies" to chocolate have been documented. It would appear that most chocolate allergies are usually linked with one of the other ingredients such as milk, peanuts and eggs or with a sensitivity to a food chemical such as caffeine, tyramine or phenylethylamine.

Maslansky and Wein reported on three people who reacted to an allergy test for chocolate using cocoa capsules. One reacted with urticaria, another with fatigue and gastric bloating and one with nausea and cramp. Only one of the three was sensitised to cocoa as detected by allergy skin testing. [1]

Merret et al tested to see if food allergy was a major cause of migraine. Their findings were that allergies could not often be detected and concluded that the food intolerance associated with migraine headaches was not related to the conventionally defined allergic mechanism—the adverse reaction was being caused by another factor such as a food chemical intolerance. [2]

Adverse reactions that have been linked with chocolate include:

Abdominal cramps and pain, Angioedema, Asthma, Bronchial complaints, Coughs, Dermatitis, Diarrhoea, Flushing, Headaches, Hypotension, Itching, Migraine, Nausea, Red ears, Rhinitis, Sneezing, Urticaria, Vomiting.

An actual intolerance or allergy to chocolate or cocoa would have to be an intolerance of either cocoa mass or cocoa butter yet these are rarely checked independently of other ingredients. Eating a chocolate bar or drinking hot chocolate is not the way to test for a "chocolate" intolerance—if you have a problem with either product it would simply mean that you could not eat that particular brand of chocolate bar or hot chocolate drink.

Intolerance problems with chocolate can be caused by any ingredient or naturally occurring chemical. In respect of ingredients it could be any of the following:

> Artificial sweeteners, butter, cocoa mass, cocoa butter, emulsifiers (usually lecithin—soya or egg), flavourings (usually vanilla—natural or man-made), grains (such as wheat, oats and rice), lactose, milk or milk powder, nuts, vegetable oils, peanuts, sugar.

In respect of a food chemical it could be any of the following:

> Caffeine and theobromine, histamine, phenylethylamine, serotonin, tyramine.

Perhaps the simplest way of testing if chocolate is a problem is to eliminate chocolate in all its forms from your diet for at least seven days. Make sure that you check all confectionery for cocoa.

If you eliminate all forms of chocolate and cocoa powder from your diet for at least seven days you will then be able to test it by first making a drink using cocoa powder, a milk and sugar or other sweetener that you know you are safe with. Make sure the cocoa powder is just that and does not contain any additional ingredients.

If you are free of any adverse reactions then you may wish to try your usual chocolate—if there is a problem then the ingredients will provide you with a list of suspects to test more fully. It is not unusual for people to react adversely to flavourings that are artificial such as vanillin.

If you find that you seem to be okay with chocolate and then your symptoms reappear it is probably worth checking the information on the different food chemicals as the problem could be as a result of a build up.

Corn

See also: *Grains.*

Corn is an increasing problem as it has now crept into a large number of processed foods so, although you may eat no actual corn, your diet could in fact be very high in it. Speer listed corn amongst the top ten allergens[3]. It has been linked with migraines[45,] and atopic dermatitis[6] in some children. Symptoms that have been reported include

> Anaphylaxis, Angioedema, Breathing problems, Dermatitis, Diarrhoea, Hives, Itching eyes and nose, Low blood pressure, Migraines, Mouth swelling.

It is a problem that is now being noticed in young children as it is found in products designed for babies. Although increasing numbers of people report having problems with corn it is still not accepted as being a major allergen by many doctors. If you have a sensitivity to corn it is a mute point as to whether it is an allergy or an intolerance as both effectively require the same treatment—avoidance.

There is little evidence to suggest cross-reactivity between corn and other cereals[7] but it has been noted that rice and corn antigens do show some similarities.[8] Because of its versatility, corn has crept into many products and, depending on your degree of sensitivity, they may all need to be avoided. You would need to avoid anything that contains the words "corn" or "maize". Check all processed foods, including sweets and candies, as corn appears in products ranging from sweets to processed meats.

All of the following either do or could contain corn, always check the label carefully and if full details are not give, as in the case of "starch" then err on the side of caution:

> Baking powder, cakes and pastries, candies, caramel flavour, cereals, chewing gums, corn, corn alcohol, corn extract, corn flakes, corn flour, corn meal, corn oil, corn starch, corn syrup, dextrin, dextrates, dextrins, dextrose, flavour enhancers, flavourings, fructose, glucose, grits, HVP, hydrolysed corn, invert sugar or syrup, maize, maltodextrin, malt syrup, marshmallow, modified starch, mono and di-glycerides, MSG, polenta, powdered sugar, processed meats, ready meals, starch, tacos, tortillas, vegetable oil, vegetable protein

The easiest way to begin testing for a corn sensitivity is to eliminate it entirely from your diet, in all its forms, for at least five days and then to eat some in the most natural form you can find. If you have had an improvement in your symptoms do beware of an unpleasant reaction when testing—you may be safest having an allergy test before attempting to eat any. If, on testing, you have no immediate symptoms then continue to add more corn-based foods into your diet stopping immediately if there is a reaction.

It is quite possible to be able to tolerate some corn but some individuals cannot tolerate any corn at all. If you fall into this group then please be aware that corn finds its way into many non-food products and that sensitivity can take place from both inhalation, ingestion and contact.

Some of the non-food products that may contain corn include:

Adhesive on stamps and envelopes, Aspirin, Bath and body powders, Cartons that are used for fruit juices and milk, Cosmetics, Cough syrups, Medicines, Ointments, Paper cups and plates, Plastic wrap, Soap, Suppositories, Toothpaste, Vitamin C, Washing powders.

Check all the products that you use—if need be contact the manufacturer to find out for certain. The symptoms caused by these forms of corn contact are wide ranging: For example Crippa and Pasolini found allergic reactions to the corn-starch powder used as glove-lubricant-powder, symptoms included breathing difficulties, rhinitis, angioedema, and asthma.[9]

If you find that you have improved greatly and then seem to have started to get ill again do not suspect that you have developed a new problem. Before you embark on any new tests double and triple check everything that you use, corn creeps into so many products that it can take quite some time before you have wholly identified all the sources that you come into contact with. Note also that corn can appear in alcoholic drinks including some beers and wines.

Eggs

Reactions to eggs are quite common, especially amongst children. Reported symptoms include:

> Allergic rhinitis, Anaphylaxis, Angioedema, Asthma, Catarrh, Dermatitis, Diarrhoea, Gastrointestinal symptoms, Hives, Migraine, Nausea, Oral allergy syndrome, Respiratory difficulties, Urticaria, Vomiting.

Rowntree et al found that 65% of children with persistent eczema and respiratory tract symptoms had a problem with eggs.[10] Guariso[11] found that for some migraine sufferers the trigger food was eggs, as did Egger.[12] Langeland in a study of eighty four children allergic to eggs, found that pruritis and exacerbations of atopic dermatitis were the most common symptoms.[13]

It has also been associated with inhalation of tame bird dander and known as "bird-egg syndrome". Maat-bleeker et al present the case of a woman who developed an egg allergy as a result of inhaled allergen sensitisation from a parrot.[14] Mandallaz et al suggest that "bird-egg syndrome" is to do with the individual developing a sensitisation to egg-yolk livetins.[15]

Although egg intolerance has often been associated with children, it can arise at any age. Egg allergens are well known with those in egg white often being the most common. Holen and Elsayed identified ovalbumin as the most allergenic portion of egg white, followed by ovomucoid, ovotransferrin and lysozyme.[16] Allergies are also possible to the proteins in egg yolk.

Problems with eggs can arise at any age. Unsel et al describe the case of a fifty-five year old woman who experienced repeated episodes of eyelid and lip swelling; itching of the throat, ears and eyes; redness and watering of the eyes; hoarseness, shortness of breath, wheezing, and coughing. The episodes began when she was fifty-three and had resulted in many visits to the emergency department. The cause was only identified when the women herself realised that the symptoms appeared soon after she ate egg or egg-containing products such as cake or pastry. Allergy tests confirmed that she did have an allergy to egg.[17]

Celakovská et al report on the case of a woman who at fifty-three developed severe atopic eczema. Allergy testing confirmed that one of the problem foods was egg. She had not experienced any problems with egg when younger but the allergy identified at age fifty-three was still present six years later.[18]

If you have always eaten eggs you will not know if they are causing you a problem. There is a much repeated story that well illustrates this point. Dr Rinkel suffered from chronic catarrh, fatigue and headaches. As his symptoms got progressively worse he began to follow advice on dietary changes and tested eggs by eating six in quick succession—rather than a worsening of symptoms he felt better.[19]

The key factor in this case was that Dr Rinkel had been eating lots of eggs each day over a long period of time. Later he eliminated eggs completely from his diet. Within a couple of days he began to feel better. On the fifth day he ate a piece of cake and fell unconscious. The cake had, of course, contained eggs. Dr Rinkel went on to become a leading allergy specialist.

The easiest way of assessing egg intolerance is to remove egg in all its forms from the diet for at least four days and then test. Avoiding eggs means avoiding it in all its forms, as whole egg, egg white, egg yolk, powdered or dry egg, so check sauces, cakes and all processed food. The following terms may also indicate the presence of egg:

Albumin, Apovitellin, Binder, Coagulant, Emulsifier, Globulin, Lecithin, Livetin, Lysozyme, Mayonnaise, Meringue, Natural flavourings, Ovalbumin, Ovomucoid, Ovaglobulin, Ovomucin, Ovomucoid, Ovotransferrin, Ovovitellin, Seasonings, Vitellin.

Products to check carefully include:

Baked goods, baking mixes, breakfast cereals, cakes, creamy fillings, egg noodles, fat substitutes, french toast, batters, bouillon, candy, custard, ice cream, soufflés, sherbets, lemon curd, macaroni, malted drinks, marshmallows, processed meat and fish products, puddings, salad dressings, sauces, soups.

The severity of egg sensitivity varies. Some people are at serious risk from anaphylactic shock and must avoid egg in all its forms, others can eat small amounts of egg, for example, in baked goods. Should you find you only react to hard boiled eggs I suggest you read the section on the naturally occurring food chemical *Tyramine*.

Eggs creep into a range of foods and other goods and may not always be listed. For example:

* In some countries, including Japan and Switzerland, lysozyme is used in medications.

- The egg used could have been in such small amounts that the manufacturer is not obliged to list it as an ingredient as may be the case with a glazing agent on baked goods. Freemont et al found lysozyme was an unlabeled additive in cheese preparation .[20]

- Egg components may also, according to Steinman, be found in cosmetics, shampoos and medications.[21]

Some points to note:

- Intolerance can be of the whole egg, egg white or egg yolk.

- Some studies have found that egg is less allergenic when cooked.

- Many vaccines are based on egg—check with your doctor before agreeing to any injection.

- It is also possible to react to other bird eggs. Langeland found cross-reactivity between hen egg white and that of turkey, goose, duck and seagull.[22]

- Many egg intolerant people can quite safely eat chicken but others experience problems.

Fish

Reactions to seafood are not uncommon and usually occur within six hours of eating. Shellfish in particular have been found to cause problems with shrimp being considered a highly allergenic food. Sicherer identifies shellfish and fish as one of the most common foods that causes problems for both children and adults.[23]

The type of fish available to you will, to a large extent, be determined by where you live. You should know that reactions have been recorded for most varieties. For example, Pascual et al, in a study from Spain, found that fish allergy was present in 22% of all people with a diagnosis of food hypersensitivity. They looked at the allergenic significance of the type of fish most commonly eaten in the area which were flatfish such as sole and hake. They found hake to be the most allergenic.[24]

Symptoms range from mild to life-threatening. Even tiny amounts of fish substances can trigger a reaction in some people. Symptoms can include:

Anaphylaxis, Bloating, Brain fogging, Breathing difficulties, Hives, Itching, Light headedness, Nasal congestion, Nausea, Stomach problems ranging from heartburn to diarrhoea, Wheezing.

Oehling et al found that the most frequent skin manifestation of fish intolerance was atopic dermatitis.[25] In a study of forty eight people with crustacean allergy, the most frequent cause of symptoms was shrimp (thirty three cases) followed by squid (twenty four cases). The most frequently found symptoms were:

Urticaria/angioedema (39 individuals),
Asthma (18 individuals) and
Rhinitis (14 individuals).[26]

It is possible to misinterpret a reaction to fish, such as tuna and mackerel, as an allergy when it might be due to a histamine sensitivity (see the section on *Histamine*). It is also possible to react to another ingredient in a fish product and so misdiagnose the cause of the problem: for example, Asero presented the case of a nineteen-year old man who experienced several episodes of angioedema of the penis and scrotum within two hours of eating canned tuna. The angioedema was found to be due to tartrazine that had been added to the tuna.[27]

Some people react solely to shellfish, any fish with high levels of histamine, or any single type of fish whether it be salmon, trout, cod, hake, herring, tuna, swordfish and so on. In a study, by Bernihisee-Broadbent et al, of people allergic to fish a number of double blind challenges to different fish species were carried out. Most of those in this study were found to be able to safely eat a different species of fish than the one they were allergic too.[28]

Other studies have, however, shown that cross-reactivity does take place.[29] Tanaka et al found reactions often took place to groups of fish and they classified seafood allergens into four groups:[30]

Salmon, sardine, horse mackerel and mackerel.
Cod and tuna.
Octopus and squid.
Crab and shrimp.

Hansen et al set out to test cross-reactivity of four species of fish—cod, mackerel, herring, and plaice—in adults with codfish allergy. Reactions were found to take place to all four types of fish and their study suggests that cross-reactivity to different fish species in adults with cod fish allergy exists, and that cod, mackerel, herring and plaice share a common antigenic structure.[31]

DeMartino et al found that some individuals with a codfish allergy could tolerate other species of fish but were more likely to react to the other species than those with non-fish allergies.[32]

Chen et al outlined the case of a forty-two year old woman who experienced itching wheals, flushing, abdominal cramps, bronchospasm, and shock approximately thirty minutes after eating kingfish (Spanish mackerel) caviar salad. She developed acute respiratory failure and profound shock. She had previously experienced acute urticaria after consuming shrimp, but did not recall any problems related to fish, milk, or chicken egg. Testing revealed that the anaphylactic reaction the woman experienced was to the kingfish caviar.[33]

They note that roe is an extremely rare cause of anaphylaxis and only one case of Russian Beluga caviar-induced anaphylaxis and one case of salmon caviar-induced anaphylactic shock have been reported in the literature pre 2009.

As fish is one of the foods that tends to provoke a very quick reaction it is unlikely that you would need to carry out any test unless you suspect histamine may be a problem or you eat fish every day. If you suspect histamine—follow the guidelines in that section. If you eat fish every day then try eliminating it from your diet for seven days to ascertain if there is a problem. Arrange for an allergy test under medical supervision.

Avoiding fish is not too difficult as it rarely creeps into non-fish dishes but do take care in restaurants where cross contamination is possible especially if the same oil is used for frying fish as well as other products such as potatoes. If you are only allergic to one form of fish you also need to be careful when eating out in case there has been cross contamination or substitution.

Shellfish, in particular, may appear in a variety of dishes and a waiter may not always be aware of their presence—ask him to check with the chef.

Lin et al gave details of a four-year old boy who had an anaphylactic reaction whenever he contacted food prepared with fish. His symptoms included intense itching in the throat and eyes, generalised urticaria, facial angioedema, coughing, wheezing and dyspnea. He reacted to several different types of fish including cod, tuna, salmon, trout, and eel, also to chopsticks contaminated with fish preparations. They suggest that the best treatment for fish allergy is avoidance which may also have to include avoiding inhalation of cooking vapours.[34]

Monti et al describe the case of a child allergic to fish who reacted with facial urticaria and angioedema after a kiss.[35]

Fruit

Any fruit can cause problems. Skin rashes, as often seen with strawberries, are a common reaction but by no means the only one. Other symptoms can include itching and swelling of the mouth, tongue and lips, and breathing problems.

It is possible to be sensitive to any individual fruit, to a number of fruits or to one of the naturally occurring chemicals found within fruit. One indicator that may help you identify a problem with fruit is seasonal fluctuation of symptoms. Do you always get rashes in the summer months? And, if yes do you at the same time eat large amounts of any of the summer fruits?

If you eat a lot of dried fruits then you could be sensitive to sulphites or salicylates—check out the respective sections. Problems with a range of fruit and vegetables is most likely to indicate a sensitivity to salicylates so if you suspect that you are reacting to a range of fruits then do please read the section on *Salicylates* before testing any individual fruit. You may find it useful to know that the only fruits that are very low in salicylate are peeled pears and bananas.

Citrus fruits contain high concentrations of chlorogenic acid which has been thought to be responsible for allergic type reactions. If you know you have a problem with any one citrus fruit you might want to consider eliminating them all for a few days and then testing. You would need to avoid all the following: clementine, grapefruit, lemon, lime, mandarin, orange, pomelo, satsuma, tangelo.

If you suspect a single fruit or summer fruits then eliminate them accordingly for at least four days and test by eating them in their most natural state which means fresh not tinned, frozen or cooked. If you do have problems with some fruits and experience an improvement in symptoms and then, later, have a return of symptoms check whether your problem is in fact one of salicylate sensitivity.

All fruits have at some point been implicated in negative reactions. Two and a half hours after eating red currants a forty-seven year old woman had symptoms including generalised urticaria, dysphagia, dyspnoea, pruritis of the palms and soles, hypotonia, and tachycardia.[36]

Oranges have been implicated in migraines[37] although this could be as a result of a tyramine sensitivity. Zhu et al report that oranges are considered to be common allergenic fruits in China. They analysed the allergic histories of twenty six orange sensitive people. Their analysis suggested that clinical symptoms of some orange-allergic subjects were different from other fruit allergies but similar to nut and other oil plant seed allergies. Interestingly they found the major allergenic components of orange reside in orange seeds instead of orange juice.[38]

Urticaria and colitis have been noted as reactions after eating papaya.[39] The oral allergy syndrome has been found to be provoked by bananas.[40] Ortoloni detected pear allergy in 22% of those with hay fever and oral allergy syndrome after eating fruit.[41] Kleinheinz et al reported on the case of a nineteen-year old woman who experienced two allergic reactions five to fifteen minutes after drinking fruit juice. Testing identified that the culprit in the fruit juice was dragon fruit.[42] Raap et al describe the case of a twenty-six year old man who developed itchy skin, urticaria, severe swelling of his lips and tongue and breathing problems within fifteen minutes after eating lychee.[43]

A French study identified ten cases (nine women, one man) of severe mango anaphylaxis.[44] A twenty-five year old man developed severe swelling of his lips, a cold sore on the inside of his lower lip, swelling of the face, and red patches on his face and ears. He had previously experienced two episodes of poison oak dermatitis. Mango contact allergy was diagnosed—he had used his teeth to peel a mango on each of the two previous days.[45]

Damian et al present four instances of Pomegranate allergy:

> A nineteen-year old man who experienced angioedema of the upper lips and tongue. The symptoms appeared a few minutes after eating fresh pomegranate.

> A thirteen-year old boy who had an episode of widespread urticaria and angioedema of the lips after ingestion of the fresh fruit.

> A thirty-one year old woman who experienced an episode of urticaria within twenty minutes eating fresh pomegranate.

> A twenty-three year old woman who complained of an episode of angioedema of the face and lips, itching of the throat, abdominal pain, and widespread urticaria, which developed approximately an hour after eating pomegranate fruit.

The reactions were confirmed as allergies using skin prick testing.[46]

Think of a fruit and someone, somewhere, will have had a negative reaction to it.

There have also been recorded instances of cross-reactivity with pollen. Ortoloni et al found cross-reactivity with almond, cherries, peaches and birch pollen in individuals with an identified birch pollen allergy.[47] Dreborg and Foucard found an association between apple, potato, carrot and birch pollen.[48] Anderson and Dreyfus found that some ragweed sensitive individuals experienced itching within the mouth when eating melons and bananas.[49]

Kim and Hussain examined the prevalence of food allergy in one hundred and thirty seven latex allergic people. They identified forty nine potential allergic reactions to foods in 21.1% of the people. The foods responsible for those reactions included:

Apple, apricot, avocado, banana, carrot, cherry, kiwi, loquat, peach, strawberry, tomato, and watermelon.

The reactions included:

Anaphylaxis, Angioedema, Asthma, Diarrhoea, Local mouth irritation, Nausea, Rhinitis, Urticaria, Vomiting.

They were unsure as to whether there was cross-reactivity or not.

Other studies have found strong links between latex allergy and certain foods most notably fruits. Brehler et al noted cross-reactions with avocado, banana, chestnut, fig, kiwi, mango, melon, papaya, passion fruit, peach, pineapple and tomato.[50] These findings have been confirmed by others.[51,52] It is also possible that anyone with allergic reactions to these foods could possibly go on to develop a sensitivity to latex.

There have been few reported cases of fig allergy and those that have been reported have been linked with cross-sensitisation to weeping fig. Antico et al found that oral allergy syndrome to fig followed by respiratory symptoms can be present in individuals not sensitised to weeping fig or having the latex-fruit syndrome. They confirmed that different parts of the fig can have different allergenicities and called for improved commercial fig extracts to be used for the diagnosis of this type of allergy.[53]

Trehan and Meuli note that mango contact allergy is more common in those with a history of poison ivy and poison oak dermatitis—these plants are closely related and mango sap contains the same uroshiol allergen.[54]

Grains

See also *Corn, Gluten, Wheat.*

The grain most likely to cause you food intolerance depends on where you live. For example, in Europe wheat is a common problem and buckwheat is often recommended as an alternative, whereas in Japan buckwheat is a major food intolerance problem. These population-based problems arise as a result of the frequency with which any one food is eaten.

Any symptom could be related to a grain sensitivity. Aside from diagnosed coeliac conditions, grains have been particularly linked with digestive system problems (bloating, abdominal pain, diarrhoea, constipation) and skin complaints.

Please note that it is a common misconception that an intolerance to cereals is always indicative of coeliac disease. In their study, Kaukinen et al found that intolerance to cereals is not a specific sign of overt or latent coeliac disease.[55]

Links between alcoholism and food intolerance, especially grains, have been found. The difficulties in giving up alcohol for some people have been misread as a problem with alcohol when in fact the problem has been with a grain. Intolerance of any food can lead to overwhelming cravings and when a product, like an alcoholic drink, contains a number of ingredients then it is not always possible to know, without thorough testing, which ingredient it is that is causing the problems. Wheat and corn have been particularly implicated in this way.[56]

Rasanen et al explored the role of cereal allergy or intolerance in children with atopic dermatitis. On oral provocation, eighteen children exhibited a positive response to wheat, three to rye, one to barley, and one to oats. Cereal-induced symptoms were dermatologic, gastrointestinal, or oropharyngeal, and their onset after provocation was immediate in eight cases and delayed in fourteen cases with one experiencing both immediate and delayed reactions. They also concluded that there was little direct link between cereal allergy and coeliac disease.[57]

Other symptoms that have been reported include:

Anaphylaxis, Angioedema, Behaviour changes, Cloudy thinking, Depression, Fatigue, Irritability, Joint pain, Muscle cramps, Skin rashes, Tingling numbness in the legs.

There are some that argue our bodies have never adapted to grains and that we should as a matter of course exclude them from our diet. The theory behind this argument is that our bodies were never designed to deal with cereals. The diet of our stone-age ancestors certainly did not include grains—they did consume carbohydrates but obtained these from fruits and vegetables. Our dependence on grains arose when settled agriculture developed and they are now an accepted part of our diet and even appear very high on the list of "healthy" foods that we should be eating.

Sadly, for some people this type of reliance on grains leads to a host of unwanted symptoms that can go undetected throughout their lifetime. A condition known as carbohydrate intolerance has also been noted and a diet excluding these used to be the main treatment for coeliac disease before the discovery of the role of gluten.[58]

If you find that you are reacting to a number of grains you may like to try a grain free diet for a few weeks and see if that helps. Certainly a spell on a grain free diet will be an education for anyone willing to try it. For some people the changes have been dramatic whilst others find they cannot manage on this type of diet. Remember that you are unique so don't expect something that works for some people to necessarily work for you. If you are a vegetarian or vegan you would not be advised to try this type of diet as you may not be able to obtain sufficient protein for your body's needs.

The biggest hurdle to living with a grain sensitivity is that we live in societies that place so much focus on carbohydrate but, as many are discovering, a diet low in carbohydrates can be extremely beneficial. If you suspect a grain sensitivity you need to eliminate that grain in all its forms from your diet for at least five days before testing. You may find a reduction in some of your symptoms or a general sense of well being.

How you react on testing the grain will probably determine whether you then continue to include it in your diet or not.

It is often thought that if you have a reaction to one grain then others are often also a problem, this is not necessarily the case. Jones et al explored the degree of intra botanical cross-reactivity among cereal grains and related grasses with the aim of better defining the prevalence of multiple grain hypersensitivity. One hundred and forty five people with cereal and/or grass allergies were involved in the study, 80% had reactivity to only one grain so don't assume that just because one grain is a problem for you that all the others will also be a problem.[59]

To test for a grain sensitivity, exclude all foods containing the grain you are testing for at least seven days and then eat it in its most natural form. Testing of grains should always be in their simplest forms—make something at home.

Don't eliminate a food without thorough testing. Wheat and other cereals are at their most nutritious in whole grain form but it is possible to be intolerant of whole grains and yet be quite comfortable with their more refined counterparts. So, if you find yourself unable to eat, for example, whole-wheat then test an organic white flour. I am suggesting an organic flour used in a simple product such as a pancake as this will eliminate the risk of misreading a test—a white loaf will contain preservatives, raising agents and may have been treated with bleaching agents all of which can give rise to problems.

Problems have been reported in respect of all grains and pseudo grains. Some examples are given below. For information on wheat, corn, or gluten please see the individual entries.

Rice

Rice has often been seen as one of the least allergenic foods but it can nevertheless cause some people serious problems. A study in France found that 17% of five hundred and eighty people with adverse reactions to food were sensitive to rice.[60]

A study in Finland of sixteen wheat sensitive children with atopic dermatitis found that 67% were also sensitive to rice.[61] Lezan et al reported on the case of a woman with rhinoconjuctivitis, asthma and urticaria as reactions to rice.[62]

Symptoms have included asthma, atopic dermatitis, contact urticaria, diarrhoea, eczema, and vomiting. Adults appear to be six times more likely than children to be sensitive to rice.[63] Two studies confirmed rice allergy as the cause of rhinitis and asthma in some individuals.[64,65]

González-Mendiola et al linked a case of asthma to the inhalation of vapours from boiling rice.[66] Nambu et al identified rice powder inhalation as the cause of a seven year old girl's asthma and rice powder, used in the making of rice cakes, as the cause of her conjunctivitis. They also found that eczema in a three-year old boy was caused by eating rice.[67]

If you have a problem with rice then do try it in various forms—you may find that whilst white rice is okay you cannot eat brown rice, can tolerate rice noodles but not rice cakes and so on.

Barley

Barley can cause problems when eaten or when the dust is inhaled. It is also a cereal that is often used in the production of alcoholic drinks such as beer and can be the "allergic" ingredient when an adverse reaction is experienced.[68]

Exposure to dust from barley has been implicated in breathing problems and skin complaints amongst farm workers.[69] Atopic dermatitis in one child was found to be caused by barley.[70]

Oats

A man who sneezed continuously for more than three decades, eventually discovered that he had a mild oat allergy.[71]

Exposure to oat dust has been implicated in breathing problems and skin complaints amongst farm workers.[72]

Atopic dermatitis in one child was found to be caused by oats.[73] The use of oats in ointments and creams is beginning to cause problems for some people—DePaz et al report on the case of a seven-year old girl who developed urticaria from a cream that was being used to alleviate her dermatitis. Testing established that the problem ingredient was oats.[74]

Some individuals with irritable bowel syndrome were found to have a sensitivity to oatmeal.[75]

Rye

Atopic dermatitis in three children was found to be caused by rye.[76] Rye is often studied alongside wheat and often not separated out as an allergen in its own right yet Baker's asthma has been found to be caused by only rye flour in some individuals.[77,78]

Buckwheat

Buckwheat is often substituted for grains as it is not taxonomically related to wheat and other cereal grains but it is not without problems. Occupational exposure to buckwheat flour has been associated with rhinitis, conjunctivitis, contact urticaria, and occupational asthma.

Davidson et al present a case of an individual developing urticaria and hypotension after eating buckwheat. Like all foods, it can cause problems for some individuals. They did find that there appeared to be no cross-reactivity between buckwheat and wheat.[79]

Varga et al note that buckwheat is known to cause severe anaphylactic reactions in susceptible adults but that it is rarely seen in children. They report on the case of a seven-year old boy who developed a grade III anaphylactic reaction after eating a cake that contained buckwheat flour. IgE testing confirmed that the boy was allergic to buckwheat.[80]

Herbs and spices

It is easy to forget about herbs and spices when assessing food intolerance but given their frequent use and the fact each is chemically complex and different they cannot be ignored. It is possible to be intolerant of any herb or spice or even a group of them. Spices in particular can cause respiratory problems when inhaled.

Virtually all herbs and spices have, at some time, caused someone problems. A few examples follow:

> Kauppinen et al identified twelve people who reacted to parsley with urticaria and angioedema.[81] A young woman experienced acute rhino conjunctivitis, facial swelling, itching in the mouth and ears, and red itchy palms and soles within five minutes of eating potatoes with a sauce containing parsley and sweet oil. Testing showed that parsley was the culprit.[82]

> A seventeen-month old boy developed urticaria, conjunctivitis, facial swelling, and a severe cough immediately after eating venison prepared in a marinade containing a variety of spices. Testing confirmed allergies to cayenne and black pepper.[83]

> Benito et al tested for reactions to various herbs. They found positive reactions to oregano, thyme, hyssop, basil, marjoram, mint, sage and lavender.[84]

> Reider et al report on instances of allergic reactions, including anaphylactic shock, to camomile and suggest that the incidence and risk of camomile allergy has been

underestimated. Some individuals with a sensitivity to camomile were also sensitive to mugwort and birch pollen.[85] Andres et al report on the case of a thirty-eight year old man who experienced severe anaphylaxis with urticaria, breathing problems and swelling within one hour after drinking camomile tea. Allergy tests confirmed that the trigger was camomile.[86]

Rhinoconjunctivitis and gastrointestinal problems were experienced as reactions to aniseed.[87]

Miller et al[88] presented fourteen cases of cinnamon-induced stomatitis and Siqueira et al presented the case of a fifty-three year old man with allergic inflammation in his mouth that was found to be caused by cinnamon in chewing gum.[89]

Ebo et al describe the case of an individual who worked in a spice factory. He had to be treated for anaphylaxis after a meal that contained coriander. He also demonstrated urticaria, angioedema, rhino conjunctivitis and broncho-spasm during handling coriander and fenugreek. On testing he was found to be allergic to both coriander and fenugreek.[90]

Gonzalez-Guitiernez et al presented the case of a patient allergic to the spice anis.[91]

Aziz and Dioszeghy describe the case of a woman who developed extreme swelling on one side of her tongue and ulceration after eating mint chocolate. The culprit was identified as being the mint in the chocolate.[92]

Chiu and Zacharisen give details of what they believe to be the first case of confirmed dill allergy. The patient developed oral pruritis, tongue and throat swelling, urticaria, vomiting and diarrhoea after eating foods cooked with dill. The person concerned also experienced reactions after smelling food prepared with dill.[93]

If you use a lot of herbs and spices in your cooking and, after having tried other tests, are still experiencing problems then consider trying a week free of them all. Then introduce them one at a time to see if there is any noticeable reaction. It would be impossible to list all the components of each herb and spice, even if they were all identified, so we are left with an "eliminate it and see" approach.

Should you find that you react to a number of herbs and spices then I suggest you try the low salicylate diet just in case you are in fact salicylate intolerant. Some of the more common herbs and spices are listed below:

Anise, basil, bay, borage, cardamom, caraway, camomile, chilli, cinnamon, clove, coriander, cumin, curry powder, dill, fennel, fenugreek, ginger, marjoram, mustard, nutmeg, oregano, paprika, parsley, pepper, peppermint, rosemary, sage, tarragon, thyme, turmeric, vanilla.

If you do find yourself sensitive to any herb or spice check labels of all processed foods and beware those that use the terms "spices" or "seasonings" as these two terms could indicate the presence of the herb or spice you are trying to avoid. It may also be necessary to check products such as toothpaste, medications, supplements and toiletries—it is surprising how many herbs and spices crop up in somewhat unusual places.

Legumes

See also *Lectins, Peanut, Saponins, Soya.*

All members of the legume family have been found to cause food intolerance symptoms. However, it is not the case that because you cannot tolerate, say, haricot beans, that all the others will also be a problem. The two main types of legumes are:

> Those that we know as common foods such as peas, beans, soya and peanuts.

> Those whose seeds or gum are used as thickeners and stabilisers in prepared foods such as locust bean gum from the carob tree.

Peanut and soya, two of the most commonly known allergens, are members of this food family and they are given sections of their own.

Legumes are an important source of protein and their consumption is very frequent in the Mediterranean region and in some Asian and African countries. In some of these regions, lentils and chickpeas are one of the main food allergens. In India legumes are the most important allergy.[94] Lentils seem to be the most common legume implicated in paediatric allergic children in the Mediterranean area.[95]

Darco et al tell us about three individuals who developed asthma and rhinitis after exposure to raw but not cooked green beans.[96] Ewan describes the case of an individual so sensitive to peas that even sitting at a table with people who were eating peas induced periorbital oedema.[97]

Orhan and Karakas report on a case of a seventeen-year old boy who had four episodes of exercise-induced anaphylactic reaction after eating lentils and two episodes of anaphylaxis after eating chickpeas.[98]

Legumes are also used as food additives due to their emulsifying properties and can be present in many manufactured foods. These hidden food allergens have the potential of causing adverse reactions in anyone with a legume sensitivity.

Gums also cause problems and cannot be ignored. Lagier et al found occupational rhinitis and asthma to guar gum amongst workers in pharmaceuticals and carpet manufacturing. One of these individuals, after eating ice cream and salad dressing containing guar gum experienced angioedema.[99] Danoff et al reported on a case of anaphylaxis after eating a hamburger containing tragacanth gum. [100]

There is a significant degree of cross-reactivity among legumes, the clinical relevance of which seems to be dependent on the dietary habits in different communities. In Spain, the consumption of several legumes is frequent and, therefore, clinical allergy to more than one species in children is common. Clinical manifestations include skin, digestive and respiratory symptoms.[101] Some of the most common legumes are listed below:

Acacia gum, adzuki bean, alfalfa, black eyed bean, black turtle bean, borlotti bean, broad bean, butter bean, cannellini bean, carob, chick pea, fava bean, fenugreek. flageolet bean, garbanzo bean, green bean, guar gum, gum arabic, haricot bean, lentils—all forms, lima bean, liquorice, locust bean gum, masur bean, mung bean, navy bean, pea, peanut, pinto bean, red kidney bean, snap bean, soya bean, string bean, tragacanth gum, wax bean, white bean.

One clear way of knowing if you have a problem with legumes is if you have ever changed to a vegetarian or vegan diet and at the same time seen an increase in health problems. The occasional attack of flatulence does not count!

One of the reasons that legumes seem to cause problems is because of their high lectin content. Lectins are carbohydrate binding proteins present in many plants. One of the legumes with a very high concentration of these is the red kidney bean. See the section on *Lectins* for further details. If you are going to eat beans please make sure you follow the guidelines for soaking and cooking very carefully. This could minimise your risk.

The only way of checking for a legume sensitivity is to eliminate them all from your diet and then test them individually. It could be that you eat very few so the test will not take very long but if you are a vegan or vegetarian the process could be lengthy and the results could have serious repercussions for your diet. Eliminate the chosen legume for at least five days and then test it in a simple meal—not a processed food.

Anybody needing to avoid all legumes will also need to check foods for gums that may have been produced from legumes. The gums currently allowed for use as food additives in the EU are listed below. They do not all come from legumes but, if you have a problem with one of them, it is probably worth removing them all and then, if you feel the need, trying some foods that contain the others over a period of time—the reason being that we do not know which chemical, protein or substance is the actual problem and it may be found across the range of gums that have a similar structure or function within food.

E410 Locust bean gum
E412 Guar gum
E413 Tragacanth
E414 Acacia gum (gum arabic)
E415 Xanthan gum
E416 Karaya gum
E417 Tara gum
E418 Gellan gum

Margarine

Margarine is not a natural food product yet, over the last few decades, has come to be seen as healthier than butter. If you are intolerant of butter then this may very well be the case but if you are not then take a close look at margarine before continuing to use it.

Margarine is a complex processed product. Not only does it contain a number of ingredients, the oils that are used have been chemically changed by the process that converts the oil to an acceptable spreadable product. The process of hydrogenation changes not only the physical form of the oils, but also alters the way they are metabolised by the body. The structure of the fatty acids is altered, or destroyed, and you are often left with trans fatty acids which are definitely not good for the body. So if you want to eat margarine avoid one that uses hydrogenated oils. This, however, is not the end of the potential problems.

Despite popular belief, margarines vary enormously in content from each other in the following ways: the types of oil used (some now do declare which oils are used but many don't), the type and number of preservatives used, the use of artificial and, so called, "natural" colours, and the quality and source of the added vitamins.

It is possible to be intolerant of one of the oils being used or of one of the preservatives the oil was treated with before being converted into margarine. You could have a problem with one of the added preservatives. Do not be lulled into assuming that a natural colour is necessarily any safer than any other—if you are sensitive to it then it will cause you a problem. The added vitamins may have been treated with preservatives and you will not know which ones.

A further difficulty with some margarines is that some contain milk products which, of course, could cause problems for anyone with a milk intolerance.

It is quite likely that during other tests you have already either excluded margarine or changed brands. If this is the case and you are symptom free then no further testing will be necessary. If you are still having problems quite simply remove margarine from your diet and do not replace it with butter for at least seven days. If there is improvement but it is slow in taking place then do not test it for at least another seven days. (It can take time for the accumulated preservatives to diminish in their impact on your body.)

Testing is straightforward—use some of your usual brand and wait and see. If no immediate reaction takes place then use it more regularly and closely monitor your health. If the brand you have been testing is a problem then choose another brand but make your choice carefully—go for the most natural and the one with least number of ingredients.

Whether you change brands, switch to butter or stop using any form of spread will depend on how you have responded to the tests.

If you find yourself intolerant of them all then don't despair—alternative spreads such as nut butters are available and oil can be substituted for butter and margarine in many forms of baking.

Meat and poultry

See also *Amines, Moulds, Nitrates.*

Meat has become the main source of protein for many people but it is not without its problems. Like any food, it is possible to be intolerant of any one meat but it is also possible to misinterpret meat problems due to naturally occurring food chemicals and additives in processed meats. There is little point in testing meats you have an aversion to or never eat unless your diet is so restrictive that you need to find foods you can incorporate.

If there is a single meat that you eat every day then consider testing it as it may be masking an intolerance problem. Also, if your diet is very high in meat products and you have health problems then you may want to consider a period without meat or with a lot less meat. Although high protein/low carbohydrate diets work for some, others need low protein/high carbohydrate diets.

It is possible to react to all forms of meat from a single animal or just to certain parts. It is possible to have a sensitivity to one meat only or to more than one. As always, it depends on the individual.

Llatser et al tell us of a woman who reacted with anaphylaxis to pork gut and kidney but was able to tolerate pork meat.[102] Hjorth and Roed-Peterson found a range of symptoms in people sensitive to beef including contact urticaria in people handling beef; and chronic diarrhoea, migraine and stomach ache after ingestion.[103]

Kelso et al found that some individuals who are allergic to one form of bird meat, such as chicken, turkey, dove or quail, may also be allergic to others including game birds.[104] Ayuso et al found cross-reactivity between beef, venison, lamb and milk and they suggest that pork rather than lamb should be included in hypoallergenic diets.[105] It is not always the case that if you are allergic to beef that you will also have problems with milk or vice versa.

A twenty-one year old woman suffered from chronic recurrent dermatitis on her lower arms. Her symptoms were always worse in the evening and during the night, and reduced noticeably over weekends. When on holiday, her dermatitis completely cleared within seven days. Various tests were carried out and eventually the culprit was found to be salami skin—the woman worked in a delicatessen store where she regularly cut and sold salami sausages.[106]

A twenty-year old man experienced itching, facial hives, lip swelling, heartburn, problems with swallowing and breathing difficulties fifteen minutes after eating chicken.[107] A forty-two year old woman with a history of occupational inhalant allergy to pork developed rhinitis, asthma, and conjunctivitis thirty minutes after eating chicken. Skin tests were positive to chicken meat.[108]

Reactions to beef have been implicated in a range of conditions. For example:

Jenkins et al found that food allergy was a major cause of infantile colitis; beef was a problem for one of the children studied.[109]

In a study of twenty seven people with chronic diarrhoea of unknown origin, Read et al found that, for one person, the cause was an allergy to beef.[110]

Lagrue et al found links between certain foods and idiopathic nephrotic syndrome (kidney disease)—one of these foods was beef.[111]

Grant found that for some migraine sufferers the triggering food was beef.[112]

Fiocchi et al estimated that beef allergy has an incidence of between 3.28% and 6.52% among children with atopic dermatitis, and may be as much as 0.3% in the general population.[113]

Allergies to raw beef have been identified amongst meat workers, usually leading to contact dermatitis.[114]

Cross-reactivity with milk has been noted[115] and Ayuso et al found cross-reactivity between beef, venison, lamb and milk.[116]

Different forms of cooking can also affect the degree of sensitivity. For example, Werfel et al found that some of those allergic to beef were able to tolerate well-cooked beef but not medium-rare and rare beef and suggested that specific IgE antibodies to heat-labile beef proteins could be the reason.[117]

To test for a meat intolerance remove all products containing the meat you are testing from your diet for at least five days. Then eat some of the meat in its most simplest form—if there is no reaction then try it in a different form. For example: if you test beef as roast beef, then try it as steak and then try it as mince.

Monitor your reactions—the method of cooking alters the chemical make-up and you may be able to eat it in one form but not another. It is not an uncommon mistake to assume that you have a problem with meat when in fact the problem lies more in the form you are eating it in. Processed meats are far higher in natural (and manmade chemicals) than, say, a joint roasted in its own juices. Grilling, stewing, barbecuing and frying all increase the amine content of meat If you suspect a problem with meat check the section on *Amines.*

The complexity of processed foods can give rise to misleading diagnoses. For example, sausages will contain many ingredients other than meat. A negative reaction does not necessarily mean a problem with the meat, the reaction could be caused by any one of the ingredients.

Continuing with the above example, caseinates are often found in sausages which, if you are milk intolerant, could cause problems. The spices in sauces and some processed meat products such as salamis can also lead to a wrong diagnosis. A reaction to these foods could indicate a salicylate sensitivity.

If you eat meat choose to eat it in its simplest form

Milk

Problems with milk are extremely common. Milk contains a number of proteins, such as casein, that can lead to allergies. Milk also contains lactose which many people cannot digest and this also leads to problems.

Lactose is the sugar in milk and it requires the enzyme lactase to digest it. Lactose intolerance is quite common and some have suggested that it arises because we were never intended to consume milk after infancy. There are tests available to identify both milk protein allergy and lactose intolerance—your doctor will be able to advice on these if you wish to find out more.

For many the relief obtained from a milk free diet is so extensive that they simply give up all forms of milk. Milk is in fact not a natural food. It is produced by females for their young and was never intended as a food for those beyond infancy. Do you know of any animal that habitually drinks the milk of another animal especially when it is grown up?

The main symptoms linked with milk problems are recurring digestive problems such as excessive gas, bloating, cramps, pain, diarrhoea, constipation, and recurring catarrhal problems. It has also been linked with:

Arthritis, Asthma, Chest complaints, Colds, Dermatitis, Ear problems, Hyperactivity, Irritability, Learning difficulties, Migraine, Sinusitis, Sleep disorders.

Rousquet et al reported that between 7 and 29% of asthma sufferers have a milk sensitivity. They also found it was often a cause of rhinoconjuctivitis in young children and may be implicated in serious otitis media.[118] Elimination diets worked for migraine sufferers in a study by Mylek and the food most usually implicated was cow's milk.[119]

Kahn et al in a study of one hundred and forty six children referred for sleep disturbance identified fifteen whose sleep problems were resolved within five weeks of starting a diet free from cow's milk. In a subsequent challenge, the sleep disturbances returned within four days of reintroducing the cow's milk.[120]

In children the two major symptoms that appear early on are gastrointestinal upsets and dermatitis. Some children appear to grow out of a milk allergy but some don't. James and Sampson found that those who retain a sensitivity to milk often have a decrease in skin disorders but an increase in gastrointestinal and respiratory symptoms.[121]

To test for a milk sensitivity avoid all milk, foods made from milk, and foods that contain milk products. Give yourself at least five milk free days before testing. If you can manage it, live without milk for two weeks and experience the effects fully.

Milk causes many people problems solely because it is consumed many times every day. Giving yourself a holiday from it will be an interesting, and hopefully, beneficial experience.

If milk has been causing you problems, the good news is that you should notice an improvement quite quickly. If your symptoms disappear or if you test and have a negative reaction then decide on a strategy:

As some people are sensitive to the chemicals the cow has ingested or been treated with, it is always safest to start your test with an organic milk. If you find you have a problem, your options are:

♦   to give up milk completely,

♦   test various products to see what you can tolerate (for example, you may be able to eat yoghurt and cheese but not drink milk; milk in baked products may be okay but not on its own; evaporated milk may be okay but not whole milk) or

♦   find out if your problem is lactose intolerance and take digestive enzymes to help if you wish to continue with milk.

What you decide to do will depend in part on how addicted to milk you are, not so much physically but by habit. At the outset giving up milk seems very strange and awkward because it seems to be everywhere and even your daily tea and coffee has to taste different. All of these problems can be overcome but it does take time to make the adjustment. Unless you have an allergic response to milk, there is nothing wrong with testing out how much milk in its different forms you can tolerate. If your unpleasant symptoms return this will provide you with the motivation you need to give it up completely.

You can try alternative milks such as goat and sheep—some people can tolerate these, others can't. There are also soy, nut, rice and oat milks now available. Initially you may find these unpalatable (your taste buds are still expecting cow's milk) but you will soon adapt or learn to do without.

Soya milk is often used as a substitute for cow's milk and was considered safe for children intolerant of milk. This is no longer thought to be the case. Lee and Heiner found that about one-fourth of those sensitive to cow's milk went on to become allergic to soy protein.[122] Various alternatives exist—

check with your doctor as to which is the safest option for your child.

Reactions to cheese only may indicate a sensitivity to food chemicals such as tyramine and histamine rather than to milk—see the section on *Amines*.

If you need to avoid milk in all its forms, the foods and ingredients you need to avoid will probably include:

> Milk in any form including dried milk, butter, buttermilk, casein, caseinate (all forms), cheese, cream, curds, custard, ghee, hydrolsates, ice cream, lactalbumin, lactose, milk chocolate, natural flavouring, rennet, sour cream, whey, white chocolate, yoghurt.

Gern et al reported casein as a cause of allergic reactions for some individuals who had been eating so called "non-dairy" products.[123] Casein and caseinates appear in a wide range of processed foods as they are used as extenders and tenderisers and, also, to nutritionally fortify certain foods so check labels carefully. They can be found in foods ranging from meat and fish products, coffee whiteners, salad dressings and bakery glazes.

Meats purchased from deli counters can pose a problem arising from cross contamination if cheese and other milk products are stored and/or sliced nearby. Bread, cakes and pastries from bakeries or bakery counters in large stores are generally not required to have ingredients labels—before buying any item that does not carry a label, check with a member of staff whether the item is milk free. To be 100% safe you would need to do this every time you make a purchase as ingredients do change.

You will need to carefully check any processed food including:

Meats and breads, desserts, and margarine.

Non-dairy products including ice creams.

Sweets and any snack foods.

Beware also of the terms "emulsifier" and "protein" as these may be milk based.

Brown sugar flavouring, caramel flavours, and high protein flour may all indicate the presence of milk protein.

Many people are very concerned about a milk free diet for fear of not getting sufficient amounts of calcium. It is quite possible, as vegans have proved, that the body's calcium requirements can be met from other foods. Foods that are high in calcium include canned salmon with bones, sardines, greens, broccoli, and tofu. You can also ask your doctor if you should take a calcium supplement.

If you are lactose intolerant and want to continue using milk you may have some options to total avoidance although this will depend on the degree of your sensitivity:

- Digestive enzymes could help.

- Some people can tolerate small amounts of lactose such as that found in ½ cup of milk.

- Foods containing lactose are sometimes better tolerated if eaten with other foods.

◆ It is possible that you can tolerate cooked milk products but not, for example, milk on your cereal.

◆ Eating smaller amounts of lactose food over a day rather than one single large amount may be easier for you.

◆ You may be able to eat some products like yoghurt without difficulty.

It will be a case of experimentation until you find the level that is acceptable to you—balancing any occurrence of symptoms with the amount and type of milk that you eat.

Peanut

See also *Lectins, Legumes.*

Peanut allergy is a serious and usually a life-long allergy affecting both children and adults. Sicherer identifies peanuts as one of the most common foods that causes problems for both children and adults.[124] It is essential that individuals with peanut allergy avoid even the slightest exposure to peanuts to prevent life threatening reactions. One of the commonest manifestation of peanut allergy is acute hives (or urticaria) following exposure.

Some people develop severe swelling and breathing problems leading to anaphylaxis. Deaths from peanuts have been reported. Some individuals are so sensitive that they will develop symptoms if they kiss someone who has eaten peanuts or eat out of a food utensil which has been in contact with peanuts. This is why many products now carry the warning that there may be traces of peanut—this means that the same machinery has been used to make the product you are buying as well as for one containing peanuts.

It had been thought that peanut oil was safe for those allergic to peanuts but some studies have identified the allergen within these oils and hence it could pose a serious problem for some individuals.[125,126]

The majority of peanut sensitive individuals are not allergic to tree nuts such as pecans, walnuts or almonds but some will have multiple sensitivities that may include tree nuts. A study by Loza and Brostoff found that 50% of individuals allergic to peanuts reported allergic reactions to other nuts as well.[127] Ewan's study of sixty two people varying in age from eleven months to fifty-three years found peanuts to be the commonest cause of allergy (47 cases), brazil nuts came in second (18 cases), followed by almond (14 cases) and hazelnut (13 cases).[128]

Multiple allergies appeared progressively with age with the commonest symptom being angioedema. Ewan concluded that children with peanut allergy are at increased risk of developing allergy to tree nuts. Interestingly only four of the sixty two reacted to other legumes (peas, lentils, beans and soya) and one of these did not react to peanuts.

Peanut allergy has rather over shadowed lesser problems. It is quite possible to be intolerant of peanuts without being allergic or at risk of anaphylaxis. However, because of the potential risks I am not advocating a peanut test at home. If you suspect peanuts as a problem please discuss testing with an allergist or doctor. If an allergy test is negative and you still believe that peanuts are a problem then eliminate them from your diet and test them but still ensure that someone is present who understands what needs to be done in case of anaphylaxis (this advice is based on the fact that allergy tests are not always 100% reliable).

Avoiding peanuts is not totally straightforward as the oil, in particular, is used in a variety of oriental dishes. It is essential that you check labels extremely carefully. Peanuts and peanut derivatives can also be found in biscuits, breakfast cereals, ice cream, soups, and sweets. Beware the terms "flavouring" and "vegetable oil". Restaurant meals and takeout meals also need to be treated with extreme caution. Remember that staff when checking ingredients may make assumptions that ingredients such as "vegetable oil" are safe.

Non-food hazards can also present themselves especially in the form of body and massage oils; watch out for the terms peanut or arachis oil. Words to look out for include:

Arachis oil, groundnuts, mixed nuts, monkey nuts, peanut, peanut butter, peanut extracts, peanut flour, peanut oil, vegetable oil.

Also, be suspicious of natural flavouring and hydrolysed vegetable protein (HVP).

The types of food that peanuts appear in include:

Baked goods, cereals, chilli, chocolate bars, crackers, egg rolls, frozen desserts, Indian food, kebabs, marzipan, spaghetti sauces, soups, sweets.

Seeds and nuts

Nuts and seeds present a hidden danger for many. Because of their versatility they are found in a wide range of processed foods and restaurant meals including meat dishes, breakfast cereals, sweets, spreads, sauces and desserts. Sicherer identifies tree nuts as one of the most common foods that causes problems for both children and adults.[129]

Nut and seed allergies usually present in childhood but intolerance can develop at any time especially as they are now, often inadvertently, consumed in greater and more regular quantities. A sensitivity to more than one could indicate a more general problem with salicylates and/or amines.

All varieties of seeds and nuts have at some time been implicated in a food intolerance or allergy problem. Reactions to nuts and seeds have included:

Abdominal cramps, Anaphylaxis, Angioedema, Breathing difficulties, Coughing, Dermatitis, Diarrhoea, Eczema, Facial swelling, Gastrointestinal problems, Hypotension, Rhinoconjuctivitis, Tingling in the mouth, Urticaria, Vomiting.

Guariso found that some young people's migraines were triggered by hazelnuts.[130] Ewan's study found allergies to brazil nut alone, brazil nut plus other nuts, almond, almond plus other nuts, hazelnut, hazelnut plus other nuts, walnut, cashew nut.[131]

Sicherer et al in a study of those with peanut and tree nut allergies found that out of one hundred and twenty two people:

Sixty eight had reactions only to peanut.

Twenty to only tree nuts.

Thirty four to both .

Of those reacting to tree nuts, thirty-four had reactions to one nut, twelve to two nuts, and eight to three or more nuts. The most common tree nuts to cause reactions were walnut, pecan and almond. Eighty nine percent of the reactions involved the skin (urticaria, angioedema), 52% the respiratory tract (wheezing, throat tightness, repetitive coughing, dyspnea), and 32% the gastrointestinal tract (vomiting, diarrhoea).[132]

Coconut has been implicated in skin problems.[133] Allergy to coconut was identified in a three-year old boy—he experienced abdominal pain, vomiting, oral allergy syndrome, and swelling of the eyelids immediately after oral contact with a coconut sweet. One year later, after eating a small portion of fresh coconut, he suffered sudden abdominal pain, vomiting, oral allergy syndrome, and swelling of the eyelids.[134]

Like the pistachio nut, the cashew nut contains oleoresins similar to those found in poison ivy and oak which can lead to contact dermatitis, stomach problems and other allergy type symptoms. The problems seem to manifest more in adults than in children. Meysman et al describe how one individual experienced severe anaphylaxis, angioedema, hypotension and shock after eating yoghurt and muesli. Investigations identified that the near fatal allergic reaction was caused by a pine nut allergy.[135]

Cross-reactivity between tree nuts and other foods and pollens have been recorded. Eriksson et al found coconut hypersensitivity in twenty two (out of three hundred and eighty) birch-pollen allergic individuals and 26% reported reactions to walnut. In respect of hazelnuts, they found those with birch-pollen allergy more often reported hypersensitivity to hazelnuts (53%) than those without pollen allergy (7%).[136]

Vocks et al found the degree of cross-reactivity among kiwi, sesame seeds, poppy seeds, hazelnuts, and rye grain was found to be very high in the people studied but the degree and exact type of cross-reactivity varied.[137]

Eating large amounts of hazelnuts can lead to an increase in nickel intake which potentially could lead to aggravating symptoms usually identified by the individual as being caused by nickel.[138]

Caubet et al describe three cases of severe snack seeds allergy in children:

A six-year old girl experienced oral itching, swelling of the lips and face, vomiting, and breathing problems within five minutes after eating a handful of sunflower seeds.

An eleven-year old boy experienced an anaphylactic reaction within a few minutes after eating pumpkin seeds.

A seven-year old boy experienced two episodes of generalized urticaria and facial swelling and a third episode with angioedema, wheezing, and acute breathing difficulties within fifteen minutes after repeatedly consuming small amounts of sunflower seeds.[139]

I don't know whether nuts and seeds are potentially more allergenic than other foods but, because of the large number of reported cases of anaphylactic shock, I do not recommend testing nuts and seeds when on your own. If you suspect nuts or seeds are a problem please discuss testing with an allergist or doctor. If an allergy test is negative and you still believe that some nuts and/or seeds are a problem then eliminate them from your diet and test them but ensure that someone is present who understands what needs to be done in case of anaphylaxis (this advice is based on the fact that allergy tests are not always 100% reliable)

Some of the more common nuts and seeds:

> Almond, brazil, cashew, coconut, hazelnut (or filbert), macadamia, pecan, pine, pistachio, poppy seed, pumpkin seed, sesame seed, sunflower seed, sweet chestnut, walnut.

You can eliminate and test each nut and seed separately or eliminate them all and then introduce them one by one during the testing phase. Remember that reactions to more than one of those high in amines or salicylate could indicate a much more general problem. Those that are particularly high in these are noted below (full details can be found in the relevant chapters).

> Those high in salicylate are almonds, brazil nuts, desiccated coconut, macadamia nuts, pine nuts, pistachio, sesame seeds, walnuts.

> Those high in amines are brazil, hazelnut, pecan, and walnut.

Sicherer et al found that accidental ingestions are common and occur most frequently outside of the home. Some of the ways in which accidental ingestion took place were as a result of:

Sharing food
Hidden ingredients
Cross contamination.[140]

Particular attention needs to be drawn to sesame seeds as allergic reactions to sesame seeds in the west have become increasingly commonplace since their introduction into processed food including burgers at many fast food outlets and the increase in the number of "exotic" meals now being eaten both in restaurants and as ready-made meals.

Anaphylaxis, angioedema, atopic dermatitis, allergic rhinitis, and bronchial asthma have all been caused by sesame seeds. Other reactions are possible and, even, likely. Remember that these vary from individual to individual. My husband, on testing sesame seeds experienced a total high which a few hours later had changed into overwhelming feelings of depression, fuddled thinking, tiredness and overall ill health. Until that time he had not known that sesame seeds caused any problems. It took more than three days for the symptoms to abate.

If sesame seeds are a problem, extreme vigilance is needed with processed and restaurant food as sesame can often be a hidden ingredient. Kagi and Wuthrich reported on a case of anaphylaxis that was caused by sesame seed in a falafel burger.[141] Food cooked in oil must always be suspected as reactions including anaphylaxis have been reported from sesame oil.[142,143]

Sesame oil finds its way into other products such as ointments and absorption through the skin can also lead to problems. Sesame oil, as a constituent of a zinc oxide liniment, was found to be the cause of contact dermatitis in fifteen out of ninety eight people with leg ulcers who had been using the liniment.[144,145]

Malten found in one hundred cases of leg ulcers, eleven people showed positive patch test reactions to a paste containing 40% sesame oil and a higher proportion showed positive reactions to 100% sesame oil.[146]

Soya

Reactions to soya have become more widespread mainly due to the increasing use of the soya bean in processed food. If you are shaking your head and saying you never eat any—check the foods you most commonly buy that are pre-prepared especially bread. Soya, and the emulsifier lecithin, are commonly used in processed foods ranging from soups to chocolate, and most mass produced bread contains soya. For many it truly is a hidden problem.

It is easy to be blasé about the safety of ingredients that appear to play a very small role in a food such as soy lecithin in bread but the reality is that soy lecithin has caused an anaphylactic reaction in a child[147] and so, for some people, is potentially very dangerous.

A thirty-eight year old man developed an anaphylactic reaction with flushing, generalized urticaria, conjunctival redness, and breathing problems three hours after eating cold Chinese noodles. He had avoided natto for the previous year as he had once experienced anaphylactic reactions half a day after eating natto. Skin prick tests were strongly positive for natto and the soup of cold Chinese noodles. The tests were also positive for poly gamma-glutamic acid (PGA), which is a major constituent of natto mucilage, an ingredient of the noodle soup.

The man was diagnosed with late-onset anaphylaxis to PGA contained in natto and the cold Chinese noodle soup. The delayed reaction was thought to be due to a delayed absorption of PGA which has to biodegrade to peptides sufficiently small enough to be absorbed in the bowel. Inomata et al note that PGA has recently been applied to a wide range of fields such as foods, cosmetics, and medicine and that anyone with a sensitivity to PGA of natto should avoid not only natto but also other materials containing PGA.[148]

Sensitivity to soya has led to cases of asthma, rhinitis, urticaria, angioedema, and digestive problems.[149] The symptoms experienced will vary from individual to individual but all of the following have been noted:

> Abdominal pain, Acne, Anaphylaxis, Angioedema, Anxiety, Asthma, Bloating, Breathing difficulties, Colitis, Conjunctivitis, Dermatitis, Diarrhoea, Eczema, Heart palpitations, Hives, Hypotension, Itching, Lethargy, Mouth sores, Rhinitis, Urticaria, Vomiting, Wheezing.

In the last few years there has been much publicity about the health benefits of soya. You should know that some researchers now believe that soya products increase the risk of thyroid disease and suggest that only small amounts are eaten.

To test for a soya sensitivity you need to eliminate it from your diet in all its forms for at least five days and then test it in its most natural form. Food terms that indicate the presence of soya include:

> Edamame beans, HVP, lecithin, miso, natto, shoyu sauce, soy bean sprouts, soya flakes, soya milk, soya protein, soy sauce, soya flour, tamari, tempeh, tofu, TVP, yuba.

You also need to avoid foods containing vegetable oil that do not state which oils are used.

Some people can tolerate soya oil but as cases of anaphylaxis have been reported it is best avoided.[150] Watch out for hidden soya, including lecithin, in processed foods. This requires very diligent label checking as it is found in so many foods—never assume something is safe. The following terms may also indicate the presence of soya:

> Bulking agent, emulsifier, flavourings, hydrolysed vegetable protein (HVP), protein, protein extender, stabiliser, starch, textured vegetable protein (TVP), thickener, vegetable broth/protein/stock, vegetable starch, vegetable gum.

If you find you only react to fermented soya products you may in fact have an amine sensitivity rather than one to soya (see the section on *Amines*).

One of the hardest aspects of a soya sensitivity is avoiding the hidden soya so if you find you are very sensitive you will need to check and double check all foods not prepared by yourself—do not trust anyone else to check for you.

Like many other foods, soya is also present in many non-food items. If you are very sensitive to soya these may also cause you a problem. Steinman lists some possible non-food sources of soya including:

> Adhesives, blankets, body lotions and creams, dog food, enamel paints, fabrics, fabric finishes, fertilisers, flooring materials, lubricants, paper, printing inks, soap.[151]

Falleroni and Zeiss report on a case of a six-year old boy who reacted to soy bean dust from a bean bag.[152]

Sugars and sweeteners

Sugar is primarily used as a sweetening agent in the form of sucrose. It is probably the most overused food in the Western world. Not only does it appear in soft drinks and sweets but is now commonly found in sauces, yoghurts, low-fat meals, tinned vegetables and processed meat products. The amount we consume without realising it is frightening.

Blood-sugar problems have frequently been linked with the over consumption of refined cereals and sugar. Other problems are also quite possible. Grant found that for some individuals migraines were caused by cane sugar.[153] Sugar intolerance can lead to:

> Anxiety, Depression, Food cravings and over eating, Hyperactivity, Irritability, Migraines, Mood swings, Nervous tension, Pre Menstrual Syndrome.

If you have any of the above symptoms and fuel your energy needs with sugary foods then try a sugar free diet for a couple of weeks and see what happens—the changes can be dramatic. Sugar has been blamed for a lot of ills which may not be justified. It is quite possible that problems that seem to have been caused by sugar have in fact been caused by other ingredients.

It is rare that we eat sugar in its most natural form and if you look at the ingredients in shop bought candies, sweets, and confectionery you will invariably find a number of food additives especially colours which have been linked with problems such as hyperactivity.

To test for a sugar problem eliminate it in all its forms. Don't be tempted to replace it with other sweeteners as these can also cause problems—avoid all sweeteners such as syrups, treacles and artificial sweeteners. You can expect to experience cravings. Make sure you plan ahead and have substitutes that you can eat such as plain crackers, crisps or fruit.

This planning aspect is vital especially if you suffer from depression as you may find the symptoms increase for a while. Treat yourself gently, rest as much as you can, take light exercise (more if able) and eat wholesome food.

Test sugar in its most natural form—simply as sugar. If you can find an organic brand choose that for preference. Avoid testing a complex product as this will not be helpful in clearly identifying a sugar problem. If you experience a sudden high and then have a change in mood for the worse—you probably have a sugar problem. It is possible that you can tolerate some sugar but you will have to experiment until you find a level that is acceptable to you.

One of the problems with sugar today is that if you read the label of any sweet biscuit, cereal, pastry, cake or candy you will find some terms other than sugar—these include glucose, syrup, fructose. Unless these originate from an accepted allergen, the source is unlikely to be mentioned. So problems can emerge for two reasons:

You can be sensitive to the food substance that the "sugar" is made from.

The way the type of sugar is metabolised by your body may not work for you giving rise to various problems.

The testing method above relates specifically to cane sugar but can be used for any type of sweetener—simply eliminate the sweetener from your diet and then reintroduce it but never substitute an alternative sweetener during the days when you are avoiding a sweetener. Some of the types of sweeteners that are readily available include.

Agave syrup, cane sugar in various forms, date syrup, fructose, glucose, honey, mannitol, maple syrup, rice syrup, sorbitol, stevia.

It seems to be the case that adding sweetness to food is always contentious whether it is seen as bad for the teeth, the cause of illnesses, or linked with obesity. What does change is the "bad guy". When I was writing the first edition of this book there was great concern over the use of the artificial sweetener Aspartame. Ten years later the spotlight is on High Fructose Corn Syrup. By the time you are reading this there may be another sweetener making the headlines.

If you use a sweetener, whether natural or not, you will need to choose the one that is best for your body and mind.

Artificial Sweeteners

In respect of artificial sweeteners, I am tempted to say don't test these just eliminate them but that is a decision you must make for yourself. My own personal concern with these is to do with their chemical complexity—my body has enough to sort out without dealing with these as well. Having said that there are very good reasons why some people need to use these type of products.

If you use an artificial sweetener and suspect that it is causing you a problem then eliminate it from your diet for a minimum of two weeks. If you find that your health is improving then prolong the length of time before trying it again. Make sure you check all sweetened items in your diet and be cautious about eating foods if you are unable to check the ingredients list.

Artificial sweeteners are manufactured products to help give you the illusion of sweetness without the calories. In many countries they have been passed as safe to eat but evidence is continually emerging of potential health problems. The most common one used is "Aspartame" which has been found to cause a diverse and bewildering array of symptoms.

Much of this evidence is anecdotal and not accepted by many but if you recognise your symptoms and know you consume large amounts of aspartame on a regular basis then you would be well advised to take the test. It is usually suggested that you eliminate all products with artificial sweeteners for a period of sixty days and monitor your health. If there is a dramatic improvement then you have probably identified the culprit. If there is no change then the choice is yours—to continue or not.[154]

Maher and Wurtman write that aspartame is consumed, primarily in beverages, by a very large number of Americans, causing significant elevations in plasma and, probably, brain phenylalanine levels. Anecdotal reports suggest that some people suffer neurologic or behavioural reactions in association with aspartame consumption. Since phenylalanine can be neurotoxic and can affect the synthesis of inhibitory monoamine neurotransmitters, the phenylalanine in aspartame could conceivably mediate neurologic effects.[155]

The reported symptoms include both physical and emotional and behavioural symptoms and these include:

Abdominal Pain, Anxiety, Bloating, Blood Sugar Problems, Brain fog, Breathing difficulties, Burning eyes or throat, Chest Pains, Chronic cough, Chronic Fatigue, Confusion, Depression, Diarrhoea, Dizziness, Excessive Thirst or Hunger, Flushing of the face, Frequent infections, Headaches/Migraines, Heart palpitations, Hives, Hypertension, Inability to concentrate, Insomnia, Irritability, Itching, Joint pains, Memory loss, Muscle spasms, Nausea, Palpitations, Seizures, Tingling sensation in limbs, Tinnitus, Urticaria, Vision problems, Weight gain.

There is a group of people who cannot safely consume aspartame. These are the sufferers of the inherited disease phenylketonuria (PKU), who are unable to metabolise the amino acid phenylalanine effectively, leading to the accumulation of potentially harmful levels. PKU is a serious, metabolic disorder, affecting 1 in 10,000 individuals and if untreated, it can cause serious brain damage.[156]

No artificial sweetener currently on the market is without drawbacks or potential health hazards. If you decide to use them then reduce the amount you consume. If you have any problems with them, or are concerned about the problems they may cause, then give them up—your body and mind will thank you. The ones currently classed as food additives in the EU are:

E950 Acesulfame K
E951 Aspartame
E952 Cyclamic acid and its Na and Ca salts
E953 Isomalt
E954 Saccharin and its Na, K and Ca salts
E955 Sucralose
E957 Thaumatin
E959 NeohesperidineDC
E 961 Neotame
E962 Salt of aspartame - acesulfame
E965 Maltitol (i) Maltitol (ii) Maltitol syrup
E966 Lactitol
E967 Xylitol
E968 Erythritol

Vegetables

See also *MSG, Salicylate, Solanine, Sulphur and Sulphites.*

Reactions to vegetables are not as well documented as, for example, reactions, to milk or nuts. This does not mean that they are "safe". The complexity of a single vegetable is immense and unwanted reactions can occur to any single vegetable or group of vegetables or naturally occurring chemical such as salicylate, solanine, sulphur and MSG found within them.

Adverse reactions to single vegetables is usually noticed early on in infancy and the vegetable is simply avoided. If you always avoid a particular vegetable then do not bother to test it unless you really feel you want to run the risk of an adverse reaction.

If you can think of a symptom then someone somewhere will probably have experienced it as a result of a sensitivity to a vegetable. Muhlemann and Wuthrich in a study of two hundred and twenty nine people with allergies found the most common food allergens to be amongst vegetables with 44.5% reacting to celery and 14.4% to carrots.[157] Quirce et al found various symptoms including bronchial asthma, urticaria and Quinckes oedema associated with a reaction to potatoes.[158]

Hoffman et al found that ten out of the twenty five eczema sufferers in their study reacted to avocado.[159] Lybarger identified respiratory, nasal and skin reactions to garlic.[160] Garlic has been linked with causing contact dermatitis and asthma.[161] Celery has been found to cause anaphylaxis, angioedema, and urticaria.[162] In a study by Mylek migraines for some individuals were triggered by cabbage.[163]

Babu and Venkatesh tested six people allergic to aubergine to establish how many parts of the aubergine were implicated. All showed positive skin prick tests to peel, pulp, raw, and cooked aubergine extracts. They concluded that aubergine has allergens in all of its edible parts with a preponderance in the peel.[164]

Tomatoes, officially classed as a fruit, yet commonly known as a vegetable are a food that is eaten widely. Unfortunately, for people with a tomato sensitivity, they are found in many processed food products. Reported adverse reactions to tomatoes include anaphylaxis, urticaria, angioedema, dermatitis, oral allergy syndrome, rhinitis, stomach problems, and asthma.[165,166,167]

Not all reactions to tomato can be classed as allergic. Tomatoes are high in a number of naturally occurring chemicals including salicylate and solanine. For some people the amount they eat simply needs to be reduced, or, for some, tomatoes need to be wholly eliminated. Reactions to tomatoes, for some people, are further complicated by cross-reactivity with latex.[168]

In thirty three people with chronic urticaria and pseudo allergic reactions to food, tests were performed with field-grown tomatoes. Seventy six percent reacted to tomato. The researchers tested for salicylates, histamine, and other components, and attributed the reactions to aromatic volatile ingredients in food, which are novel agents that elicit pseudo allergic reactions in chronic urticaria. Histamine, salicylate, and a direct mast-cell histamine release were not involved in this reactivity to naturally occurring pseudo allergens.[169]

Riffelmann and Wenzel reported on the case of one person who had three reactions within three months after eating mixed salad. The symptoms were tongue swelling and angioedema of the lips. Tests for a sensitivity to lettuce were negative but were found to be positive to rocket.[170]

The authors of a French study note that shitake mushrooms are the second most eaten mushroom in the world. In Asia, toxic adverse effects due to picking or consumption of shiitake mushrooms are well known. As consumption of these mushrooms is increasing in the West there is concern that a similar pattern may emerge. Herault et al outline the case of a seventy-eight year old woman who experienced an extensive rash, diagnosed as dermatitis, all over her body including her face and scalp. The rash appeared two days after she had eaten a large amount of raw shitake mushrooms.[171]

After eating guacamole dip with chips, a fifteen-year old boy developed coughing, wheezing, nasal stuffiness, generalized urticaria and swelling around the eyes. The reaction was treated as an anaphylactic reaction and skin testing confirmed an allergy to avocado which is the primary ingredient of guacamole. As anaphylaxis to avocado is often linked with latex sensitization, tests for latex sensitivity were also carried out but these were all negative.[172]

Cabbage is often seen as a safe food—rarely allergenic and, of course, good for you. The truth is that cabbage has been implicated in a range of health problems. Eriksson found that some adults who had an acetylsalicylic acid (aspirin) intolerance were also intolerant of other foods including cabbage.[173] In 1985, Jones et al, induced remission in twenty patients with active Crohn's disease by dietary changes. In some of these patients symptoms were found to be triggered by the Brassica family of vegetables which include cabbage, broccoli, and cauliflower.[174]

Elimination diets worked for migraine sufferers in a 1992 study by Mylek and although the food most usually implicated was cow's milk, other problem foods included cabbage.[175] Some people find they can tolerate cabbage only when cooked. In respect of food chemicals, cabbage is low in amines and salicylate, contains natural sulphur which may be a problem for someone with a severe sensitivity to sulphites, is high in naturally occurring goitrogens, and pickled cabbage is high in histamine.

The biggest problem with vegetables is that we are told they are good for us and so many of us make ourselves eat them against our own innate wisdom. If you have ever tried to eat a diet high in vegetables and have felt worse then you could have a food chemical problem. There is no easy way of suggesting where you start. Read the food chemical sections especially the symptoms and see if any spring out at you.

For example, if you have a lot of joint pain then it may be useful to try the solanine test. Alternatively, if you dislike or feel ill after eating aubergine, then the histamine test may be useful. If you have a problem with a large number of vegetables, and fruit, then consider checking for a salicylate sensitivity.

Reactions to individual vegetables, as shown above, have been reported. If you suspect a vegetable (and are sure it is not a food chemical problem) then remove it from your diet for four days and then test it. Make sure the test vegetable is fresh not frozen or tinned and preferably organic. Don't add a sauce to it.

Some people have tried eating diets high in raw vegetables and have often after an initial improvement felt much worse. This is not necessarily indicative of a sensitivity. It could be, quite simply, that your body cannot handle raw vegetables— try cooking them. The cooking process changes the vegetable and, in many cases, removes or reduces the allerginicity.

The high chemical content of vegetables can also lead to problems of misdiagnosis. It is quite possible to test a vegetable, react badly to it, eliminate it totally, feel better and a few days or weeks later experience a return of all the symptoms. If this happens it is indicating that it was not the individual vegetable but one of the chemicals—read the lists and see if you need to do a further test.

A further problem is the one-off reactions that can occur often leading to quite strong adverse reactions after eating a vegetable you are usually okay with. This is more likely to be caused by pesticide contamination. It is safer when testing vegetables to at first eat them in their organic form.

Wheat

See also: *Gluten, Grains.*

Wheat frequently causes problems mainly because we eat so much of it. It is not unusual to eat some wheat at every meal—in cereal at breakfast, sandwiches at lunch, biscuits as a snack, and pasta or bread with the evening meal. Speer[176] has wheat listed in the top ten most allergenic foods and Andre et al[177] found wheat to be one of the most common allergenic foods. Reactions to wheat tend to fall into three groups:

*   A sensitivity to gluten.

*   Intolerance of or allergy to wheat more generally.

*   Problems with whole-wheat.

If you have any stomach problems, skin problems, and/or arthritis you should consider testing wheat. Blood sugar problems, especially if your main snack foods contain wheat, could be another indicator. Wheat has also been found to cause migraines[178,179] for some people and even asthma.[180,181] Twelve per cent of one hundred and two children who were allergic to pollen were also allergic to wheat.[182]

Wheat allergy is one of the most common food allergies in children but little data is available regarding its natural history. Corinne et al studied one hundred and three children who all had a history of wheat allergy. Their main aim was to identify the length of time that the allergy lasted. They found that the rates of resolution were 29% by four years, 56% by eight years, and 65% by twelve years. Whilst higher wheat IgE levels were associated with poorer outcomes, many children with even the highest levels of wheat IgE did outgrow wheat allergy. They concluded that the median age of resolution of wheat allergy is approximately six and a half years. But, in a significant minority, wheat allergy persists into adolescence.[183]

If you have a problem with wheat do not assume that you have a gluten sensitivity. Not all problems with wheat are related to gluten. Test each of the gluten grains individually to see if you can tolerate them—there is no point in limiting your diet unnecessarily. There are now lots of cookbooks to help people with wheat and/or gluten problems so it should not pose too many problems with finding alternatives.

To test for a wheat sensitivity exclude all foods containing wheat for at least seven days and then eat it in its most natural form. Testing of grains should always be in their simplest forms—make something at home like a very simple pancake. If you test wheat in the form of bread and experience a reaction you will not know whether you are reacting to the wheat, a preservative, raising or bleaching agent.

It is possible that whilst wheat combined with yeast or other raising agent may be a problem, wheat in other recipes may be okay. Don't eliminate wheat without thorough testing. Although wheat, and other cereals, are at their most nutritious in whole grain form it is possible to be intolerant of whole grains and yet be quite comfortable with their more refined counterparts. So, if you find yourself unable to eat whole-wheat, test an organic white flour. I am suggesting an organic flour used in a simple product such as a pancake as this will eliminate the risk of misreading a test if you eat a product with a large number of ingredients.

Symptoms, even with wheat, can be dose related. Hanakawa et al reported on the case of a twenty-four-year-old Japanese woman who had suffered for two years from attacks of urticaria, breathing irregularities, and temporary loss of consciousness due to a sudden fall in blood pressure—all of which were associated with exercise after the ingestion of wheat. On testing with varying amounts of wheat in different forms they were able to identify the amounts at which reactions took place: for example, exercise following ingestion of 64g, but not 45g, of bread induced generalised urticaria for this individual.[184]

Wheat is the main ingredient or can be found in most of the following:

> Bread crumbs, bran, bulgar, cereal extract, coffee substitutes, couscous, crackers, durum wheat, enriched flour, farina, flour, gluten, gluten flour, gram flours, high protein flour, HVP, modified food starch, natural flavouring, pasta, semolina, spelt, soy sauce, starch, vinegar made from grain, wheat bran, wheat germ, wheat germ oil, wheat starch, white flour, whole wheat.

> Alcoholic beverages such as beer and whiskey.

You may find that you are only sensitive to wheat but if you find that after some respite from symptoms they begin to re-emerge you may want to consider testing other grains as some degree of cross-reactivity has been noted. For example, some individuals with wheat induced asthma also reacted to rye, barley and soya flours.[185]

If you find you are very sensitive to wheat, it is also important to check that you are not using non-food products that contain some wheat. Varjonen et al report on a case of contact urticaria caused by hydrolysed wheat in a body cream.[186] Wheat germ oil is sometimes used as a carrier oil for massage oils—to be on the safe side check all creams, ointments, lotions, shampoos, conditioners and similar products.

References

[1] Maslansky L, Wein G. Chocolate allergy: a double-blind study. Conn Med J 1971;35:5-9.

[2] Merrett J, Peatfield RC, Rose FC, Merrett TG. Food related antibodies in headache patients. J Neurol Neurosurg Psychiatry 1983;46(8):738-42.

[3] Speer F. Multiple food allergy. Ann Allergy 1975;34:71-6.

[4] Grant EC. Food allergies and migraine. Lancet 1979;1(8123):966-9.

[5] Speer F. Allergy and migraine: a clinical study. Headache 1971;11:63-67.

[6] Sampson HA, McCaskill CC. Food hypersensitivity and atopic dermatitis: evaluation of 113 patients. J Pediatr 1985;107(5):669-75.

[7] Kalverman M, Forck G. Crossreactivity between grass and corn pollen antigens. Int Arch Allergy Appl Immunol 1978;57:549-53.

[8] Hoffman D, Yamamato F, Ceiler B, Haddad Z. Specific IgE antibodies in atopic eczema. J Allergy Clin Immunol 1975;(55)256-67.

[9] Crippa M, Pasolini G. Allergic reactions due to glove-lubricant-powder in health-care workers. Int Arch Occup Environ Health 1997;70(6):399-402.

[10] Rowntree S et al. Development of IgE and IgG antibodies to food and inhalant allergens in children at risk of allergic disease. Arch Dis Childh 1985;60: 727-735.

[11] Guariso G, Bertoli S, Cernetti R, Battistella PA, Setari M, Zacchello F. Migraine and food intolerance: a controlled study in pediatric patients. Pediatr Med Chir 1993;15(1):57-61.

[12] Egger J, Wilson J, Carter CM, Tuner MW, Soothill JF. Is migraine food allergy? A double-blind controlled trial of oligoantigenic diet treatment. Lancet 1983;2:865-869.

[13] Langeland T. Allergy to hen's egg white in atopic dermatitis. Acta Derm Verereol: 1985;114(Suppl):109-12.

[14] Maat-Bleeker de F, Van Dijik A G, Berrens L. Allergy to egg yolk possibly induced by a sensitisation to bird serum antigens. Ann Allergy 1985;54:245-48.

[15] Mandallaz M, de Weck AL, Dahinden CA. Bird egg syndrome. Int Arch Allergy Appl Immunol 1988;87:143-50.

[16] Holen E, Elsayed S. Characterisation of four major allergens of hen egg-white by IEF/SDS-PAGE combined with electrophoretic transfer and IgE immunoautoradiography. Int Arch Allergy Appl Immunol 1990;9:136-41.

[17] Unsel M, Sin AZ, Ardeniz O, Erdem N, Ersoy R, Gulbahar O, Mete N, Kokuludağ A. New onset egg allergy in an adult. J Investig Allergol Clin Immunol. 2007;17(1):55-8.

[18] Celakovská J, Ettlerová K, Ettler K, Krcmová I. Food allergy to egg with the onset at adult age. Revue Française d'Allergologie 2010;50:628-633.

[19] Mackarness R. Not All In The Mind. Pan 1976.

[20] Fremont S, Kanny G, Nicolas JP, Moneret-Vautrin DA. Prevalence of lysozyme sensitization in an egg-allergic population Allergy 1997;52(2):224-8.

[21] Steinman HA. Hidden allergens in foods. J Allergy Clin Immuno 1996;98(2):241-50.

[22] Langeland T. A clinical and immunological study of allergy to hen's egg white. Allergy 1983;38:399-412.

[23] Sicherer SH. Manifestations of food allergy: evaluation and management. Am Fam Physician 199915;59(2):415-24,429-30.

[24] Pascual C, Martin Esteban M, Crespo JF. Fish allergy: evaluation of the importance of cross-reactivity. J Pediatr 1992;121(5 Pt 2):S29-34.

[25] Oehling A, Fernandez M, Cordoba H, Sanz ML. Skin manifestations and immunological parameters in childhood food allergy. J Investig Allergol Clin Immunol 1997;7(3):155-9.

[26] Castillo R, Carrilo T, Blanco C, Quiralte J, Cuevas M. Shellfish hypersensitivity: clinical and immunological characteristics. Allergol Immunopathol (Madr) 1994;22(2):83-7.

[27] Asero R. A strange case of "tuna allergy". Allergy 1998;53(8):816-7.

[28] Bernihisel-Broadbent J, Scanlon SM, Sampson HA. Fish hypersensitivity.1. In vitro and oral challenge results in fish-allergic patients. J Allergy Clin Immunol 1992; 89:730-7.

[29] Bernihisel-Broadbent J, Scanlon SM, Sampson HA. Fish hypersensitivity.1. In vitro and oral challenge results in fish-allergic patients. J Allergy Clin Immunol 1992; 89:730-7.

[30] Tanaka R, Ichikawa K, Hamano K. Clinical characteristics of seafood allergy and classification of 10 seafood allergens by cluster analysis. Arerugi 2000;49(6):479-86.

[31] Hansen TK, Bindslev-Jensen C, Skov PS, Poulsen LK. Codfish allergy in adults: IgE cross-reactivity among fish species. Ann Allergy Asthma Immunol 1997;78(2):187-94.

[32] de Martino M, Novembre E, Galli L, de Marco A, Botarelli P, Marano E, Vierucci A. Allergy to different fish species in cod-allergic children: in vivo and in vitro studies. J Allergy Clin Immunol 1990;86(6,Pt1):909-14.

[33] Chen YH, Wu HJ, Tsai JJ, Lee MF. Anaphylactic shock caused by a 33-kDa alpha S1-casein-like allergen in kingfish caviar. J Investig Allergol Clin Immunol 2009;19(3):245-246.

[34] Lin HY, Shyur SD, Fu JL, Lai YC, Lin JS. Fish induced anaphylactic reaction: report of one case. Zhonghua Min Guo Xiao Er Ke Yi Xue Hui Za Zhi 1998;39(3):200-2.

[35] Monti G, Bonfante G, Muratore MC, Peltran A, Oggero R, Silvestro L, Mussa GC. Kiss-induced facial urticaria and angioedema in a child allergic to fish. Allergy 2003;58(7):684-5.

[36] Zollner TM, Schmidt P, Kalveram CM, Emman AC, Boehncke WH. Allergy 2000;55(5):511.

[37] Egger J, Wilson J, Carter CM, Tuner MW, Soothill JF. Is migraine food allergy? A double-blind controlled trial of oligoantigenic diet treatment. Lancet 1983;2:865-869.

[38] Zhu SL, Ye ST, Yu Y. Allergenicity of orange juice and orange seeds: a clinical study. Asian Pac J Allergy Immunol 1989;7(1):5-8.

[39] CJ. Anaphylaxis to kiwi fruit and related 'exotic' items. J Asthma 1983;20:193-6.

[40] Ortoloni C, Ispano M, Pastorello E, Bisi A, Ansaloni R. The oral allergy syndrome. Ann Allergy 1988;61:47-52.

[41] Ibid.

[42] Kleinheinz A, Lepp U, Hausen BM, Petersen A, Becker WM. Anaphylactic reaction to (mixed) fruit juice containing dragon fruit. J Allergy Clin Immunol 2009 Jul 9.

[43] Raap U, Schaefer T, Kapp A, Wedi B. Exotic food allergy: anaphylactic reaction to lychee. J Investig Allergol Clin Immunol. 2007;17(3):199-201.

[44] M. Morisset, D.-A. Moneret-Vautrin, P. Beaumont, B. Bonnefoy-Guionnet, et al. Anaphylaxie à la mangue : dix cas rapportés au Réseau allergovigilance aspects cliniques et fréquence actuelle. Revue Française d'Allergologie 2010;50(4):406-409.

[45] Trehan I, Meuli GJ. Mango contact allergy. J Travel Med 2010 Jul-Aug;17(4):284.

[46] Damiani E, Aloia AM, Priore MG, Nardulli S, Ferrannini A. Pomegranate (Punica granatum) allergy: clinical and immunological findings. Ann Allergy Asthma Immunol 2009 Aug;103(2):178-180.

[47] Ortoloni C, Ispano M, Pastorello E, Bisi A, Ansaloni R. The oral allergy syndrome. Ann Allergy 1988;61:47-52.

[48] Dreborg S, Foucard T. Allergy to apple, carrot and potato in children with birch pollen allergy. Allergy 1983; 38:167-72.

[49] Anderson BL, Dreyfuss EM, Logan J, Johnstone DE, Glaser J. Melon and banana sensitivity coincident with ragweed pollinosis. J Allergy 1970;45:310-18.

[50] Brehler-R; Theissen-U; Mohr-C; Luger-T. Latex-fruit syndrome: frequency of cross-reacting IgE antibodies. Allergy. 1997; 52(4): 404-10.

[51] Beezhold DH, Sussman GL, Liss GM, Chang NS. Latex allergy can induce clinical reactions to specific foods. Clin Exp Allergy 1996;26:416-22.

[52] Blanco C, Carrillo T, Castillo R, Quiralte J, Cuevas M. Latex allergy: clinical features and cross-reactivity with fruits. Ann Allergy 1994;73:309-14

[53] Antico A, Zoccatelli G, Marcotulli C, Curioni A. Oral allergy syndrome to fig. Int Arch Allergy Immunol. 2003 Jul;131(2):138-42.

[54] Trehan I, Meuli GJ. Mango contact allergy. J Travel Med 2010 Jul-Aug;17(4):284.

[55] Kaukinen K, Turjanmaa K, Maki M, Partanen J, Venalainen R, Reunala T, Collin P. Intolerance to cereals is not specific for coeliac disease. Scand J Gastroenterol 2000;35(9):942-6.

[56] Randolph TG, Moss RW. An Alternative Approach to Allergies. Revised ed. Harper, 1990.

[57] Rasanen L, Lehto M, Turjanmaa K, Savolainen J, Reunala T. Allergy to ingested cereals in atopic children. Allergy 1994;49(10):871-6.

[58] Gottschall E. Whatever happened to the cure for coeliac disease? Nutritional Therapy Today. 1997:7(1):8-11.

[59] Jones SM, Magnolfi CF, Cooke SK, Sampson HA. Immunologic cross-reactivity among cereal grains and grasses in children with food hypersensitivity. J Allergy Clin Immunol 1995;96(3):341-51.

[60] Andre F, Andre C, Colin L, Cacaraci F, Cavagna S. Role of new allergens and of allergen consumption in the increased incidence of food sensitivity in France. Toxicology 1994;93(1):77-83.

[61] Varjonen E, Vainio E, Kalimo K, Juntunen-Backman K, Savolainen J (1995) Skin-prick test and RAST responses to cereals in children with atopic dermatitis. Characterization of IgE-binding components in wheat and oats by an immunoblotting method Clin Exp Allergy 25:1100-7.

[62] Lezan A, Igea J, Davila I, Martin JA, Alonso MD et al. Occupational asthma and contact urticaria to rice in a housewife. Schweiz me Wschr 1991;121(p2):296.

[63] Lewis WH, Imber WE. Allergy epidemiology in the St Louis, Missouri, area V. Cereal ingestants. Ann Allergy 1975;35:251-4.

[64] Kumar R, Srivastava P, Kumari D, Fakhr H, Sridhara S, Arora N, Gaur SN, Singh BP. Rice (Oryza sativa) allergy in rhinitis and asthma

patients: a clinico-immunological study. Immunobiology. 2007;212(2):141-7.

[65] Kumar R, Kumari D, Srivastava P, Khare V, Fakhr H, Arora N, Gaur SN, Singh BP. Identification of IgE-mediated food allergy and allergens in older children and adults with asthma and allergic rhinitis. Indian J Chest Dis Allied Sci. 2010 Oct-Dec;52(4):217-24.

[66] Gonzalez-Mendiola R, Martin-Garcia C, Carnes J, Campos J, Fernandez-Caldas E. Asthma induced by the inhalation of vapours during the process of boiling rice. Allergy.2003;58 :1202– 1203

[67] Nambu M, Shintaku N, Ohta S. Rice allergy. Pediatrics. 2006 Jun;117(6):2331-2.

[68] Nusem D, Panasoff J. Beer anaphylaxis. Isr Med Assoc J. 2009 Jun;11(6):380-1.

[69] Manfreda J, Holford-Strevens V, Cheang M, Warren CP. Acute symptoms following exposure to grain dust in farming. Environ Health Perspect 1986 Apr;66:73-80.

[70] Rasanen L, Lehto M, Turjanmaa K, Savolainen J, Reunala T. Allergy to ingested cereals in atopic children. Allergy 1994 Dec;49(10):871-6

[71] http://news.bbc.co.uk/hi/english/health/newsid_812000/812034.stm

[72] Manfreda J, Holford-Strevens V, Cheang M, Warren CP. Acute symptoms following exposure to grain dust in farming. Environ Health Perspect 1986 Apr;66:73-80.

[73] Rasanen L, Lehto M, Turjanmaa K, Savolainen J, Reunala T. Allergy to ingested cereals in atopic children. Allergy 1994 Dec;49(10):871-6

[74] De Paz Arranz S, Pérez Montero A, Remón LZ, Molero MI. Allergic contact urticaria to oatmeal. Allergy. 2002 Dec;57(12):1215.

[75] Triggs CM, Munday K, Hu R, Fraser AG, Gearry RB, Barclay ML, Ferguson LR. Dietary factors in chronic inflammation: food tolerances and intolerances of a New Zealand Caucasian Crohn's disease population. Mutat Res. 2010 Aug 7;690(1-2):123-38.

[76] Rasanen L, Lehto M, Turjanmaa K, Savolainen J, Reunala T. Allergy to ingested cereals in atopic children. Allergy 1994 Dec;49(10):871-6

[77] Ehrlich R, Prescott R. Baker's asthma with a predominant clinical response to rye flour. Am J Ind Med. 2005 Aug;48(2):153-5.

[78] Letrán A, Palacín A, Barranco P, Salcedo G, Pascual C, Quirce S. Rye flour allergens: an emerging role in baker's asthma.Am J Ind Med. 2008 May;51(5):324-8.

[79] Davidson AE, Passero MA, Settipane GA. Buckwheat-induced anaphylaxis: a case report. Ann Allergy 1992; 69(5):439-40.

[80] Varga EM, Kollmann D, Zach M, Bohle B. Anaphylaxis to Buckwheat in an Atopic Child: A Risk Factor for Severe Allergy to Nuts and Seeds? Int Arch Allergy Immunol. 2011 Mar 30;156(1):112-116.

[81] Kauppinen K, Kousa M, Reunala T. Aromatic plants--a cause of severe attacks of angio-edema and urticaria. Contact Dermatitis. 1980 Jun;6(4):251-4.

[82] Cordobés-Durán C, García-Menaya JM, Lombardero M, Ledesma A, Bobadilla P. Detection of a 12-kilodalton lipid transfer protein allergen in parsley. J Investig Allergol Clin Immunol. 2007;17(4):282-3.

[83] Gimenez L, Zacharisen M. Severe pepper allergy in a young child. WMJ. 2011 Jun;110(3):138-9.

[84] Benito M, Jorro G, Morales C, Pelaez A, Fernandez A. Labiatae allergy: systemic reactions due to ingestion of oregano and thyme. Ann Allergy Asthma Immunol 1996 May;76(5):416-8.

[85] Reider N, Sepp N, Fritsch P, Weinlich G, Jensen-Jarolim E. Anaphylaxis to camomile: clinical features and allergen cross-reactivity. Clin Exp Allergy 2000;30(10):1436-43.

[86] Andres C, Chen WC, Ollert M, Mempel M, Darsow U, Ring J. Anaphylactic reaction to camomile tea. Allergol Int. 2009 Mar;58(1):135-6

[87] Garcia-Gonzalez JJ, Bartolome-Zavala B, Fernandez-Melendez S, Barcelo-Munoz JM, Miranda Paez A, Carmona-Bueno MJ, Vega-Chicote JM, Negro Carrasco MA, Ameal Godoy A, Pamies Espinosa R. Occupational rhinoconjunctivitis and food allergy because of aniseed sensitization. Ann Allergy Asthma Immunol 2002;88(5):518-22.

[88] Miller RL, Gould AR, Bernstein ML. Cinnamon-induced stomatitis venenata, Clinical and characteristic histopathologic features. Oral Surg Oral Med Oral Pathol. 1992 Jun;73(6):708-16.

[89] Siqueira AS, Santos CC, Cristino MR, Silva DC, Pinheiro MG, Pinheiro JJ. Intraoral contact mucositis induced by cinnamon-flavored chewing gum--a case report. Quintessence Int. 2009 Oct;40(9):719-21.

[90] Ebo DG, Bridts CH, Mertens MH, Stevens WJ. Coriander anaphylaxis in a spice grinder with undetected occupational allergy. Acta Clin Belg. 2006 May-Jun;61(3):152-6.

[91] Gonzalez-Gutierrez ML, Sanchez-Fernandez C, Esteban-Lopez MI, Sempere-Ortells JM, Diaz-Alperi P. Allergy to anis. Allergy 2000;55(2):195-6.

[92] Aziz O, Dioszeghy C. Allergic hemiglossitis as a unique case of food allergy: a case report. J Med Case Reports. 2008 Mar 6;2:71.

[93] Chiu AM, Zacharisen MC. Anaphylaxis to dill. Ann Allergy Asthma Immunol 2000;84(5):559-60.

[94] Niphadker PV, Patil SP, Bapat MM. Legumes, the most important food allergen in India. Allergy 1992;47:318.

[95] Sanchez-Monge R, Pascual CY, Diaz-Perales A, Fernandez-Crespo J, Martin-Esteban M, Salcedo G. Isolation and characterization of relevant allergens from boiled lentils. J Allergy Clin Immunol 2000;106(5Pt1):955-961.

[96] Daroca P, Crespo JF, Reano M, James JM, Lopez-Rubio A, Rodriguez J. Asthma and rhinitis induced by exposure to raw green beans and chards. Ann Allergy Asthma Immunol 2000;85(3):215-8.

[97] Ewan PW. Clinical study of peanut and nut allergy in 62 consecutive patients: new features and association. BMJ 1996;312:1074-78.

[98] Orhan F, Karakas T. Food-dependent exercise-induced anaphylaxis to lentil and anaphylaxis to chickpea in a 17-year-old boy. J Investig Allergol Clin Immunol. 2008;18(6):465-8

[99] Lagier F, Cartier A, Somer J, olovich J, Malo J-L. Occupational asthma caused by guar gum. J Allergy Clin Immunol 1990;85:785-90.

[100] Danoff D, Linoln L, Thomson DMP, Gold P. Big Mac Attack. N Eng J Med 1978;298:1095-96.

[101] Martinez San Ireneo M, Ibanez Sandin MD, Fernandez-Caldas E Hypersensitivity to members of the botanical order Fabales. J Investig Allergol Clin Immunol 2000;10(4):187-99.

[102] Llaster R, Polo F, De La Hoz F, Guillaumet B. Alimentary allergy to pork. Crossreactivity among pork and kidney and lamb gut. Clin Exp Allergy 198;28(8):1021-5.

[103] Hjorth N, Roed-Peterson. Occupational protein contact dermatitis in food handlers. J Contact Derm 1976;2:28-42.

[104] Kelso JM, Cockrell GE, Helm RM, Burks AW. Common allergens in avian meats. J Allergy Clin Immunol 1999;104(1):202-4.

[105] Ayuso R, Lehrer SB, Lopez M, Reese G, Ibanez MD, Esteban MM, Ownby DR, Schwartz H. Identification of bovine IgG as a major cross-reactive vertebrate meat allergen. Allergy 2000;55(4):348-54.

[106] Wantke F, Simon-Nobbe B, Poll V, Gotz M, Jarisch R, Hemmer W. Contact dermatitis caused by salami skin. Contact Dermatitis 2011 Feb;64(2):111-114.

[107] González-Mancebo E, Pastor C, González-de-Olano D, Gandolfo-Cano M, Melendez A, Cuesta J, Zapatero A, Bartolomé B. Identification of allergens in chicken meat allergy. J Investig Allergol Clin Immunol. 2011;21(4):326-7.

[108] Hilger C, Swiontek K, Hentges F, Donnay C, de Blay F, Pauli G. Occupational inhalant allergy to pork followed by food allergy to pork

and chicken: sensitization to hemoglobin and serum albumin. Int Arch Allergy Immunol. 2010;151(2):173-8.

[109] Jenkins HR, Pincott JR, Soothill JF, Milla PJ, Harries JT. Food allergy: the major cause of infantile colitis. Arch Dis Child 1984 Apr;59(4):326-9.

[110] Read NW, Krejs GJ, Read MG, Santa Ana CA, Morawski SG, Fordtran JS. Chronic diarrhea of unknown origin. Gastroenterology 1980 Feb;78(2):264-71.

[111] Lagrue G, Heslan JM, Belghiti D, Sainte-Laudy J, Laurent J. Basophil sensitization for food allergens in idiopathic nephrotic syndrome. Nephron 1986;42(2):123-7.

[112] Grant EC. Food allergies and migraine Lancet 1979;1(8123):966-9.

[113] Fiocchi A, Restani P, Riva E. Beef allergy in children. Nutrition 2000 Jun;16(6):454-7.

[114] Kumar A, Freeman S. Protein contact dermatitis in food workers. Case report of a meat sorter and summary of seven other cases. Australas J Dermatol 1999 Aug;40(3):138-40.

[115] Werfel SJ, Cooke SK, Sampson HA. Clinical reactivity to beef in children allergic to cow's milk. J Allergy Clin Immunol 1997 Mar;99(3):293-300.

[116] (1) Ayuso R, Lehrer SB, Lopez M, Reese G, Ibanez MD, Esteban MM, Ownby DR, Schwartz H. Identification of bovine IgG as a major cross-reactive vertebrate meat allergen. Allergy 2000;55(4):348-54.

[117] Werfel SJ, Cooke SK, Sampson HA. Clinical reactivity to beef in children allergic to cow's milk. J Allergy Clin Immunol 1997;99:293-300.

[118] 0Rousquet J, Chanez P, Michel F-B. The respiratory tract and food hypersensitivity. In: Metcalfe DD, Sampson HA, Simon RA. (eds) Food Allergy: Adverse reactions to foods and food additives, 2nd ed. Blackwell Science 1997.

[119] Mylek D. Migraine as one of the symptoms of food allergy. Pol Tyg Lek 1992;20-27;47(3-4):89-91.

[120] Kahn A, Mozin MJ, Rebuffat E et al. Milk intolerance in children with persistent sleeplessness: a prospective double blind crossover evaluation. Pediatrics 1989;84:595-603.

[121] James JM, Sampson HA. Immunolgic changes associated with the development of tolerance in children with cow milk allergy. J Pediatr 1992;121:371-77.

[122] Lee EJ, Heiner DC. Allergy to cow's milk 1985. Pediatrics in review 1986;7(7):195-203.

[123] Gern JE, Young E, Evrard HM, Sampson HA. Allergic reactions to milk-contaminated "nondairy" products. New Eng J Med 1991;324:976-79.

[124] Sicherer SH, Burks AW, Sampson HA. Clinical features of acute allergic reactions to peanut and tree nuts in children. Pediatrics 1998;102(1):e6.

[125] Hoffman DR, Collins-Williams C. Cold pressed peanut oils may contain peanut allergen. J Clin Allergy Immunol 1994;93(4):801-02.

[126] Moneret-Vautrin DA, Hatahet R, Kanny G. Risks of milk formulas containing peanut oil contaminated with peanut allergens in infants with atopic dermatitis. Pediatr Allergy Immunol 1994;5:184-8.

[127] Loza C, Brostoff J. Peanut Allergy (review). Clin Exp Allergy 1995;25:493-502.

[128] Ewan PW. Clinical study of peanut and nut allergy in 62 consecutive patients: new features and association. BMJ 1996;312:1074-78.

[129] Sicherer SH. Manifestations of food allergy: evaluation and management. Am Fam Physician 199915;59(2):415-24,429-30.

[130] Guariso G, Bertoli S, Cernetti R, Battistella PA, Setari M, Zacchello F. Migraine and food intolerance: a controlled study in pediatric patients. Pediatr Med Chir 1993;15(1):57-61.

[131] Ewan PW. Clinical study of peanut and nut allergy in 62 consecutive patients: new features and association. BMJ 1996;312:1074-78.

[132] Sicherer SH, Burks AW, Sampson HA. Clinical features of acute allergic reactions to peanut and tree nuts in children. Pediatrics 1998;102(1):e6.

[133] Stricker WE, Anorve-Lopez E, Reed CE. Food skin testing in patients with idiopathic anaphylaxis. J Allergy Clin Immunol 1986;77:516-519.

[134] Tella R, Gaig P, Lombardero M, Paniagua MJ, García-Ortega P, Richart C. A case of coconut allergy. Allergy. 2003 Aug;58(8):825-6.

[135] Meysman M, Schelfaut D, Vincken W. A not so healthy muesli: a case report. Acta Clin Belg. 2009 Jul-Aug;64(4):366-8.

[136] Silverman K, Evans SM, Strain EC, Griffiths RR. Withdrawal syndrome after the double-blind cessation of caffeine consumption. New Eng J Med 1992;327:1109-14.

[137] Vocks E, Borga A, Szliska C, Seifert HU, Seifert B, Burow G, Borelli S. Common allergenic structures in hazelnut, rye grain, sesame seeds, kiwi, and poppy seeds. Allergy 1993;48(3):168-72.

[138] Flyvholm MA, Nielsen GD, Andersen A. Nickel content of food and estimation of dietary intake Z Lebensm Unters Forsch 1984;179:427-31.

[139] Caubet JC, Hofer MF, Eigenmann PA, Wassenberg J. Snack seeds allergy in children. Allergy 2010 Jan;65(1):136-7.

[140] Sicherer SH, Burks AW, Sampson HA. Clinical features of acute allergic reactions to peanut and tree nuts in children. Pediatrics 1998;102(1):e6.

[141] Kagi, MK; Wuthrich, B. Falafel-burger anaphylaxis due to sesame seed allergy. Lancet 1991;338: 582.

[142] Chiu, JT; Haydik, IB. Sesame seed oil anaphylaxis. J Allergy Clin Immunol 1991;88:414-415.

[143] Kanny G, De Hauteclocque C, Moneret-Vautrin DA Sesame seed and sesame seed oil contain masked allergens of growing importance. Allergy 1996;51(12):952-7.

[144] Van Dijk E, Neering H, Vitányi BE. Contact hypersensitivity to sesame oil in zinc oxide ointment. Ned. Tijdschr. Geneeskd. 1972,116:2255.

[145] Van Dijk E, Neering H, Vitányi BE. Contact hypersensitivity to sesame oil in patients with leg ulcers and eczema. Acta Derm.-Vener. 1973;53:133.

[146] Malten, KE. Sesame oil contact hypersensitivity in leg-ulcer-patients. Contact Dermatitis Newsletter 1972;(11):251.

[147] Renaud C, Cardiet C, Dupont C. Allergy to soy lecithin in a child. J Pediatr Gastroenterol Nutr. 1996 Apr;22(3):328-9.

[148] Inomata N, Chin K, Nagashima M, Ikezawa Z. Late-onset anaphylaxis due to poly (gamma-glutamic acid) in the soup of commercial cold Chinese noodles in a patient with allergy to fermented soybeans (natto). Allergol Int 2011 Mar 25.

[149] Koerner CB, Sampson H. Diets and Nutirtion. In Metcalfe DD, Sampson HA, Simon RA. Food Allergy: Adverse Reactions to Foods and Food Additives. Blackwell, 1991.

[150] Dueñas-Laita A, Pineda F, Armentia A. Hypersensitivity to generic drugs with soybean oil. N Engl J Med. 2009 Sep 24;361(13):1317-8.

[151] Steinman HA. Hidden allergens in foods. J Allergy Clin Immuno 1996;98(2):241-50.

[152] Falleroni AE, Zeiss CR. Bean bag allergy revisited: a case of allergy to inhaled soybean dust. Ann Allergy Asthma Immunol 1996;77(4):298-302.

[153] Grant EC. Food allergies and migraine. Lancet 1979;1(8123):966-9.

[154] Starr, JH. Sweet Poison. New Horizon, 2004.

[155] Maher TJ, Wurtman RJ. Possible neurologic effects of aspartame, a widely used food additive. Environ Health Perspect 1987;75:53-7.

[156] www.food.gov.uk/safereating/chemsafe/additivesbranch/sweeteners/551 74

[157] Muhlemann RJ, Wuthrich B. Food allergies 1983-1987. Schweiz Med Wochenschr0 1991;121(46):1696-700.

[158] Quirce S, Diet Gomez ML, Hinjosa M Cuevas, Rivas MF, Pujana J et al. Housewives with raw potato-induced bronchial asthma. Allergy 1989;44:532-36.

[159] Hoffman D, Yamamato F, Ceiler B, Haddad Z. Specific IgE antibodies in atopic eczema. J Allergy Clin Immunol 1975;(55)256-67.

[160] Lybarger JA, Callagher JS, Pulver DW, Litwin A, Brooks A, Bernstein IL. Occupational asthma induced by inhalation and ingestion of garlic. J Allergy Clin Immunol 1982;69:448-54.

[161] Perez-Pimiento AJ, Moneo I, Santaolalla M, de Paz S, Fernandez-Parra B, Dominguez-Lazaro AR . Anaphylactic reaction to young garlic. Allergy 1999;54(6):626-9.

[162] Ortoloni C, Pastorello E, Luraghi MT, Della Torre F, Bellani M, Zanussi C. Diagnosis of intolerance to food additives. Ann Allergy 1984;53:587-91.

[163] Mylek D. Migraine as one of the symptoms of food allergy. Pol Tyg Lek 1992;20-27;47(3-4):89-91.

[164] Babu BNH; Venkatesh YP. Clinico-immunological analysis of eggplant (Solanum melongena) allergy indicates preponderance of allergens in the peel. WAO Journal 2009;2(9):192-200.

[165] Jesenak M, Rennerova Z, Babusikova E, Havlicekova Z, Jakusova L, Villa MP, Ronchetti R, Banovcin P. Food allergens and respiratory symptoms. J Physiol Pharmacol. 2008 Dec;59 Suppl 6:311-20.

[166] Zacharisen MC, Elms NP, Kurup VP. Severe tomato allergy (Lycopersicon esculentum). Allergy Asthma Proc. 2002 Mar-Apr;23(2):149-52.

[167] 3. Vandenplas O, Sohy C, D'Alpaos V, Nootens C, Thimpont J, Weigand D, Scheurer S. Tomato-induced occupational asthma in a greenhouse worker. J Allergy Clin Immunol. 2008 Dec;122(6):1229-31.

[168] Vozza I, Ranghi G, Quaranta A. Allergy and desensitization to latex. Clinical study on 50 dentistry subjects. Minerva Stomatol. 2005 Apr;54(4):237-45.

[169] Zuberbier T, Pfrommer C, Specht K, Vieths S, Bastl-Borrmann R, Worm M, Henz BM. Aromatic components of food as novel eliciting factors of pseudoallergic reactions in chronic urticaria. J Allergy Clin Immunol. 2002 Feb;109(2):343-8.

[170] Riffelmann F, Wenzel M. Tongue swelling and angioedema due to rocket (Eruca sativa) Allergologie 2009;32(8):303-305.

[171] Herault M, Waton J, Bursztejn AC, Schmutz JL, Barbaud A. Shiitake dermatitis now occurs in France. Ann Dermatol Venereol 2010 Apr;137(4):290-293.

[172] Abrams EM, Becker AB, Gerstner TV. Anaphylaxis related to avocado ingestion: a case and review. Allergy Asthma Clin Immunol 2011 Jun 10;7(1):12.

[173] Eriksson NE. Food sensitivity reported by patients with asthma and hay fever. A relationship between food sensitivity and birch pollen-allergy

and between food sensitivity and acetylsalicylic acid intolerance. Allergy 1978;33(4):189-96.

[174] Jones VA, Workman E, Freeman AH, et al. Crohn's disease: maintenance of remission by diet. Lancet 1985;2:177-180.

[175] Mylek D. Migraine as one of the symptoms of food allergy. Pol Tyg Lek 1992;20-27;47(3-4):89-91

[176] Speer F. Multiple food allergy. Ann Allergy 1975;34:71-6.

[177] Andre F, Andre C, Colin L, Cacaraci F, Cavagna S. Role of new allergens and of allergen consumption in the increased incidence of food sensitivity in France. Toxicology 1994;93(1):77-83.

[178] Egger J, Wilson J, Carter CM, Tuner MW, Soothill JF. Is migraine food allergy? A double-blind controlled trial of oligoantigenic diet treatment. Lancet 1983;2:865-869.

[179] EC. Food allergies and migraine. Lancet 1979;1(8123):966-9.

[180] Sandiford CP, Tee RD, Newman-Taylor AJ. Identification of crossreacting wheat, rye, barley and soya flour allergens using sera from individuals with wheat-induced asthma. Clin Exp Allergy 1995;25(4):340-9.

[181] Williams AJ, Church SE, Finn R. An unsuspected case of wheat induced asthma. Thorax. 1987;42(3):205-6.

[182] De Martino M, Novembre E, Cozza G, deMarco A, Bonazza P, Vierucci A. Sensitivity to tomato and peanut allergies in children monosensitized to grass pollen. Allergy 1988;43:206-13.

[183] Corinne A. Keet MD, MS; Elizabeth C. Matsui MD, MHS; Gitika Dhillon MD; Patrick Lenehan BS; Melissa Paterakis BS; Robert A. Wood MD. The natural history of wheat allergy. Annals of Allergy, Asthma and Immunology 2009, vol. 102, no. 5, pp. 410 – 415.

[184] Hanakawa Y, Tohyama M, Shirakata Y, Murakami S, Hashimoto K. Food-dependent exercise-induced anaphylaxis: a case related to the amount of food allergen ingested. Br J Dermatol 1998;138(5):898-900.

[185] Sandiford CP, Tee RD, Newman-Taylor AJ. Identification of crossreacting wheat, rye, barley and soya flour allergens using sera from individuals with wheat-induced asthma. Clin Exp Allergy 1995;25(4):340-9.

[186] Varjonen E, Petman L, Makinen-Kiljunen S. Immediate contact allergy from hydrolyzed wheat in a cosmetic cream. Allergy 2000;55(3):294-6.

6 The Next Stage

How easily you adapt to your new diet will depend on a number of factors including:

+ The degree of improvement you've experienced.

+ How motivated you are

+ Whether you have identified all your food intolerance problems.

+ How long you were ill for and how severe your problems were.

+ How restricted your diet has become.

+ The amount of support you have.

If there has been any improvement please do not give up on yourself—keep going. One of the things that quite commonly happens is that there is some major improvement and then things seem to get a little sluggish and you start to doubt the wisdom of your new diet. Give it a chance.

The older you are the longer you have been putting your body under stress. Your body's first reaction is likely to have been one of celebration and joy and now, after the party is over, it is taking time to recover. Trust it and let it heal in its own time. If you return to your old diet you will simply set yourself back. It is possible, and very useful, to re-test foods but if you had an adverse reaction do not re-test for at least six months. Hopefully, as your body recovers it will be able to tolerate more foods over time. If an allergy has been diagnosed and the reactions you experienced were very severe your wisest course of action will be to always avoid the food.

There are cases where people find they have become intolerant of virtually all foods. I suspect that this is more to do with an undiagnosed food chemical intolerance rather than a problem with the foods themselves. However, if you find that this is happening then rotate the foods that you can eat and gradually introduce others. You rotate foods by never eating the same food on more than one day in any four day cycle.

If you have been carrying large amounts of excess weight you will have found this diminishing. If this is the case you will probably experience times of extreme hunger—do not starve your body, feed it. This seems to be part of an adjustment process and I doubt you will gain any weight. After a few days the need for extra food will subside and if you still need to lose weight it will once again begin to diminish. Avoid the temptation to speed up this process—you will only place extra stress on your body. It doesn't need it. Feed it the right foods for it, and your mind, and your weight will adjust quite naturally.

When you have identified a food intolerance problem you may want to find out more about your condition. The internet is a wonderful place for accessing this information but what you need to try avoid doing is overwhelming yourself with information. At first limit yourself to a couple of sites and gradually build up your store of information. If you want to explore the medical literature you will probably, at some point, find conflicting articles. Personally I am very wary of any articles or research, regardless of who is responsible for it, that categorically states that a particular food is not a problem or that a specific condition is never caused, or at least made worse, by food intolerance. Remember that:

- The individual doctor or researcher may have specific interests that "colour" their work.

- Research is often funded by large corporations including pharmaceutical companies and food manufacturers.

- The research may have been limited to a very small number of cases.

- Food intolerance is often simply not accepted.

- The overall evidence is clear—any food can lead to any symptom.

So search, read and discuss—information is liberating. But, in the final analysis, trust your own results from your own eliminating/testing. The only person who can help you stick to your diet is you. You can help yourself in a number of ways:

- Plan your meals—get really organised.

- Eat regularly and so avoid getting hungry and being tempted to eat the wrong foods.

- Buy cookbooks that provide you with recipes you can use and experiment with.

- Congratulate yourself on having done so well.

+ Build in treats that you know you can tolerate.

+ Make contact with others with a similar problem.

Be extremely cautious about any processed food or food prepared by others. The easiest way of getting caught out is by trusting someone who says "It's safe—I checked". Ask for a list of the ingredients and check for yourself. If this seems like overkill take note of the following case reported by Schwartz.[1]

A child with a known milk allergy was given chicken soup in a hospital and the result was a nearly fatal case of anaphylaxis. The sodium caseinate that was in the soup had not been recognised by the staff as being a milk protein. More worryingly, they had also perceived reactions to milk as relatively harmless.

Don't assume that because you understand your problems that everyone else will—they won't.

You will have setbacks—accidental ingestion of the food or substance you can't tolerate. The best advice I can give is treat yourself gently. The reaction will pass so don't give in to any cravings that might come. Eat the foods that are safe, rest and learn from the experience.

You've simplified your diet, carried out food tests using the elimination diet and are feeling better. You're quite confident that you know what causes your problem and are careful to avoid the problem foods. Then, inexplicably you have a reaction and find that, no matter how hard you think back and check the food you've eaten, there is no way in which you could have eaten one of your problems foods. You have introduced some new foods but all the ingredients listed are ones you know you are okay with. Have you found a new food problem?

It is possible but, before you put yourself through the rigors of further eliminating and testing, re-check the foods you have introduced. If any of these are processed products remove them from your diet for at least seven days and then try again. If you have a reaction again then the likely culprit is a hidden ingredient that is probably on your NO list. How did this happen? Quite simply legislation may permit a manufacturer not to list an ingredient constituting less than a specific percentage of the total product. You can, if you so choose, write to the manufacturer to verify your own results.

This was demonstrated very clearly in a report by Enrique et al in respect of eggs. They cite the instance of a twenty-five year old woman who had been diagnosed with an egg allergy and told to avoid all forms of egg protein. Two months later she experienced a further reaction after eating a strawberry and cream candy. No egg compound was stated on the candy label. Tests confirmed that it was the candy she was reacting to and also identified the presence of ovoalbumin, which is added to candies as a binder, and this was confirmed by the manufacturers.[2] Cantani reported on similar problems with milk.[3] Other possible forms of contamination are listed by Steinman including:[4]

Manufacturing plants using the same equipment to make different products such as milk ice cream and dairy free ice cream.

The use of the same oil to cook different foods.

"Natural" flavours.

Ingredient switching that involves use of a different oil, nut, sugar, herb or spice.

Binders and emulsifiers which are not defined.

The move towards wanting to eat organic food seems to arise naturally as part of wanting a healthier diet. Certainly, when one reads about the potential health problems that can be caused by pesticides it seems like the only logical step to take but is it always the right way to go? I ask this question because when no pesticides are used the plant produces more of its own natural toxins so some vegetables and fruit will at times have a higher salicylate content than those grown with the use of pesticides. I am not advocating eating non-organic food but I am raising this issue especially for anyone with a salicylate sensitivity. If you are salicylate sensitive and have found that some of your problems have become worse after switching to organic food this could be the reason why.

One of the areas I have not covered in this book is that of botanical families and the reason for this is I tend to find these mislead people. As Barnes Koerner and Sampson say "Although it is often helpful to think of foods in certain botanical families, no clinical evidence supports consistent broad intra-botanical or intra-species cross-reactivity".[5]

Sometimes the problem is misread and the true problem is in fact a food chemical one. I think the safest approach is never to assume that you will react to all members of a botanical family rather to test of each of the foods individually and if you find you react to them all then first check that you do not have a salicylate or other food chemical sensitivity.

Biochemical individuality is about far more than the foods you can tolerate. It very much deals with the amount of each nutrient that your body needs. For example, some people need far more B6 than others. To assess your individual needs on this level you would need medical help and it may not be forthcoming. Many doctors still believe that the RDA (recommended daily allowance) for vitamins and minerals is more than adequate for all and that we all need the same amounts. Others disagree strongly saying that the RDAs will simply stop the occurrence of diseases such as scurvy (lack of vitamin C) or pellagra (lack of B3).

In 1969 Linus Pauling introduced us to "Orthomolecular Medicine" which focuses on using naturally occurring substances like vitamins, minerals, trace elements, enzymes and amino acids to treat illness and maintain health. Doctors embracing this approach had some startling successes including the treatment of schizophrenia with B vitamins by Dr Hoffer and others. But, sadly this approach has never been embraced more generally by the medical profession. This is not because it does not work or is in some way flawed.

There is a great deal of evidence to indicate that existing diets do not provide adequate amounts of vitamins and minerals even by RDA standards. Werbach's[6] survey of nutritional influences on illness includes a section on nutritional deficiencies. To give you an overview of the type of problems that exist, I will summarise a selection of the findings:

- An American study found that the majority of the US population, especially adult women, were obtaining levels of calcium below the Recommended Dietary Allowance.

- Chromium deficiency is common in western diets relying on high intake of refined foods.

- Iodine deficiency is common in many countries.

- Magnesium intake is often low. Vitamin B3 is often deficient in elderly people.

- Selenium is frequently inadequate in Western diets.

- Thousands of people develop vitamin A deficiency each year.

- Vitamin C intake is often below recommended daily amounts.

- Zinc is commonly inadequate in Western diets.

There are also vitamins and minerals that can help people with food related problems. Some examples follow:

- Vitamin C can help reduce a reaction which raises the blood histamine level and may also reduce MSG sensitivity.

- Vitamin B12 may help reduce sulphite sensitivity.

- A magnesium deficiency may increase allergic reactions and lead to symptoms similar to chronic fatigue syndrome.

- Calcium supplementation may reduce allergic reactions.

- Vitamin B6 may reduce MSG sensitivity.

- A molybdenum deficiency may lead to sulphite sensitivity.

- Vitamin B3 may slow down the release of histamine.

- Vitamin B5 may reduce allergic reactions particularly those involving the nasal passages and help in cases of chronic fatigue.

Getting adequate vitamins and minerals is essential not just to maintain health but also to reduce the impact of allergic reactions on the body. Philpott says that vitamins C, B6 and B3 "have the most important value in preventing such maladaptive reactions".[7] A poor diet that doesn't provide us with the full range of vitamins and minerals that we need can also lead to illness both physical and mental. Some examples follow:

- Vitamin B1 deficiency can lead to irritability, depression, confusion, and an acute sensitivity to noise.

- Diets low in pantothenic acid can make some people depressed, withdrawn and irritable.

- Low potassium levels can lead to fatigue.

- A good quality multi vitamin and mineral supplement with additional vitamin C would seem to be essential for all of us especially if we have been ill or are getting older.

- Older readers should note that studies have shown that many older people do not absorb adequate amounts of many essential nutrients. Supplementation may be the way to remedy this.

Some links between an excess of iron and the development of cancer cells has been found which is why some vitamin companies now produce multi vitamin and mineral supplements that exclude iron. Supplements of individual vitamins and minerals should be taken with great care as many of them rely on other vitamins and minerals to be of any benefit and some in large doses can be toxic. Some examples of problems follow:

- Evening primrose oil can exacerbate temporal lobe epilepsy and may exacerbate mania.

- High doses of folic acid may decrease levels of B12.

- High doses of iron can lead to stomach problems.

- Manganese intoxication can lead to irreversible movement and other neurological disorders. It can also lead to high blood pressure in some people over forty.

- Too much selenium has been associated with hair loss, thickened, fragile nails, nausea and fatigue.

- Exceptionally high doses of Vitamin A can lead to birth defects.

- Large doses of vitamin B6 can lead to neurological symptoms.

- Very large doses of vitamin C can lead to diarrhoea.

Find out as much as you can before you supplement with single vitamins and minerals—it is generally thought that the safest option is to only take individual vitamins and minerals alongside a multi. Pregnant women should seek medical advice as some supplements can be harmful to the foetus.

Be very cautious about the preparations you buy—you really do need to look for quality and you do need to be sure that any supplement you buy is safe for you. If the label is confusing then check with the manufacturer. And if you start to feel worse after taking any supplement—stop taking it immediately. Never start taking more than one supplement at a time—if you have a reaction you will not know which supplement is to blame.

Beware of hypo-allergenic supplements as these may not be safe for you. If you feel unsure of how to go about boosting your system with vitamins and minerals consult a nutritionist and/ or read some of the very good books on the market.

Ideas for other ways in which you can boost your system follow. By making sure that you eat as much fruit and vegetables as you can you will help keep your system balanced towards alkalinity which will also help you feel better. Increase the amount of exercise you take, relax more and do things that interest you. Ill health affects all aspects of our lives and we need to start to put the balance back.

Having said that—don't go mad and try to do too much! This will over tire you and then frustrate you if you find yourself ill again. Gently build up your activities and take lots of rest. Some people have found great help from taking digestive enzymes—find out if these could help you. Various herbs, such as echinacea, can help boost the system but take them with care (reactions to herbs are not unusual) especially if you are salicylate sensitive. You may also like to consider using a water filter to reduce the amount of chlorine and other water contaminants being ingested.

In an article on the detoxification enzyme systems, Liska explores the complex process involved in the body's ongoing battle to deal with toxins. "These mechanisms exhibit significant individual variability, and are effected by environment, lifestyle, and genetic influences". Impairment of these systems could lead to the development of conditions such as Parkinson's Disease, Fibromyalgia, Chronic Fatigue Syndrome, and other immune system disorders.[8]

It has been suggested that the difficulties some individuals experience with food chemicals and food additives is due to some impairment in this detoxification system that predominantly takes place in the liver. Some individuals have seen improvement in their sensitivities as a result of using supplements to help the liver. Amongst these "cysteine", a sulfur amino acid is used by the body to manufacture glutathione which plays a vital role in the body's ability to eliminate toxins.

Also, ensure your diet is as high as it can be with fruit and vegetables as many of these, including cabbage and Brussels sprouts, encourage enzyme activity. This effect of vegetables and fruits could in part explain why they seem to protect against certain cancers. And look after your gut. The gastrointestinal tract provides a physical barrier to many unwanted products and, after the liver, is the second major site in the body for detoxification. You need to have a healthy gut so eat well and ensure that you have a good supply of healthy bacteria. If you have had gastrointestinal problems, or still have them, you may find some of the acidophilus supplements useful.

Carl Pfeiffer says that "Every thought and feeling we have can alter, and is altered by, the chemistry of our body".[9] If you have been ill for a long time and are now experiencing better health do not be surprised if, after the initial relief and joy, you experience some feelings of anger and grief about the time you have lost and that you may have been misdiagnosed for many years. By all means look at these feelings, write them out, talk them through with a friend or counsellor but do not get stuck in them

The simple truth is that although improvement in your condition may have been a long time in coming it has arrived. For many people the answer may never appear. Consider yourself lucky, focus on the positive feelings and look to the future. The past, no matter how right or wrong elements in it may have been, has now gone. As you recover, focus on the present and when you feel stronger turn your attention to the future remembering that now you are free of chronic ill health there are many things you can once again dream of doing and actually begin to do.

But please don't make the mistake of rushing into a whole range of new activities. If you were ill for a long time you need to allow yourself time to recover. Release your imagination, explore ideas, rest and try to take pleasure from the moment, the here and now. Getting healthier is an amazing experience, take the time to savour it and the fact that you have been the one to bring it about.

When you feel ready to embark on your new life be gentle with yourself. List all the things you want to do and prioritise them. Don't try do them all at once—you'll exhaust yourself. By being clear about your goals you'll achieve them more easily and with less effort. As you throw yourself into new activities do remember to take the time to monitor your diet and health. As your body and mind changes you may need to make adjustments in your diet.

You may have found yourself, rather than feeling inspired, feeling lost, cast adrift with little idea of what to do next, as if everything that seemed real and solid before has changed. This is most likely to arise if you had been having many psychological symptoms that have now improved or disappeared. The best advice I can give you is to take some time to get to know yourself.

Enjoy the process. Don't assume that just because you did something before in a certain way that you have to continue doing so. You have changed and you can now choose what you do and how you respond. You may find it useful to take some time to explore what your dreams are. A couple of brain storming exercises might help. Firstly write out fifty things you enjoy doing and then write out fifty things you really want to do. Let your imagination fly.

Remember, it was not your fault you were ill. You have always tried to do the best for yourself. Celebrate your achievement.

You may find it useful to make contact with others with a similar problem. How you do this will depend on you as an individual and also where you live. Some options include:

+ Support groups—check in your area or with a national organisation that deals with your condition.

+ On-line through discussion forums.

+ Reading books and articles. If books are out of print then ask at your library—in the UK many can be borrowed via the British lending library.

+ One to one—if you know someone else with similar problem arrange to meet regularly.

Support can also come from family, friends and work colleagues but don't expect them to understand if you don't explain it to them. Anybody who has seen you have a reaction will probably be understanding but some of those who haven't may be very sceptical and may even hinder you.

Have patience with others and do try to avoid evangelising—rather than helping this often has the effect of putting people off. I always try to remember what I was like before I knew about my food intolerance problems—basically I knew nothing about allergy or food intolerance and really wasn't very interested. You can't change others so don't be hurt if people don't follow your advice or don't believe you.

Your biggest source of support is always going to be yourself.

Nobody else can control what you eat but you. Become your own best friend and stop worrying about what anybody else thinks.

Tips and tricks

Here are a few suggestions to help make your life a little easier.

Plan your meals ahead so that you always have food available that you can eat.

Use your freezer—make up extra batches of meals for the days when you just can't be bothered.

Never trust food given to you by others unless you know for definite that they understand what your problems are. Even then you would be better to check by asking for details of the ingredients.

Prepare a list of foods that you can eat (rather than ones you can't) that you can give to others or restaurants to help them in preparing a meal for you.

If you are making a long journey always take more food with than you think you will need—unexpected delays can turn into nightmares if you don't have food and drinks with you that are safe for you.

Take time out to invent or discover new recipes—this will help you stop getting bored with the food you eat.

If you buy any processed food—ALWAYS check the ingredients as these do change.

Use the word "allergic" rather than "food intolerant" with people you don't know—allergy is more accepted and most people will understand that this means you have a problem.

Don't assume that anybody cooking for you will know what foods contain salicylates, MSG, sulphur, additives, milk, wheat etc...

Eat as balanced and varied diet as you can.

Avoid defining yourself as allergic or food intolerant (or any other label). Remain the person who you are. You are not your condition or illness.

Never forget that what works for you may not work for anyone else—avoid converting and being converted to particular diets and/or supplements.

Take advice but then check it out for yourself—nobody has all the answers. The best expert on you is always you.

If reactions affect your mind prepare to deal with them. Have strategies in place for avoiding contact, explaining your behaviour, making yourself feel safe. You may also find it useful, when well, to write yourself a note which you can read when a reaction takes hold—it should explain what is happening and reassure you that it will pass. If you have someone who understands what is happening talk to them as sometimes this helps minimise the effects of the anxiety.

Be gentle with yourself.

References

[1] Schwartz, RH. Near-fatal anaphylaxis to chicken soup and near-anaphylactic events to cow's milk occurring in the hospital. J Allergy Clinical Immunol; 1993;91(1pt2):152.

[2] Enrique E, Cistero-Bahima A, Alonso R, San Miguel MM. Egg protein: a hidden allergen in candies. Ann Allergy Asthma Immunol. 2000;84(6):636.

[3] Cantani A. Hidden presence of cow's milk proteins in foods. J Investig Allergol Clin Immunol 1999;9(3):141-5.

[4] Steinman HA. Hidden allergens in foods. J Allergy Clin Immuno 1996;98(2):241-50.

[5] Barnes Koerner C, Sampson HA. Diets and Nutrition. In: Metcalfe DD, Sampson HA, Simon RA. Food Allergy: Adverse reactions to foods and food additives, 2nd ed. Blackwell Science 1997.

[6] Werbach M R. Nutritional Influences on Illness: A sourcebook of clinical research 2nd edition. Third Line Press 1996.

[7] Philpott W H, Kalita D H. Brain Allergies: The Psychonutrient and Magnetic Connections. Keats 2000.

[8] Liska DJ. The detoxification enzyme systems. Altern Med Rev 1998: 3(3), 197-98.

[9] Pfeiffer CC. Mental and Elemental Nutrients. Keats 1975.

Final Word

We have reached the end of *The Food Intolerance Handbook*. I hope you have found the information useful and that you are well on the way to finding the ideal diet for you.

Health, after life itself, is our most precious possession. Without it we are limited and restricted in what we do and even in how we think.

Never give up on finding the answers to your health problems. Work with your doctors but remember they do not know everything and do not have all the answers.

Always do the very best you can for yourself and remember you are a unique individual.

I wish you well.

Sharla

Appendix 1: Food Additives

Food additives are substances added to a food during processing for a specific purpose such as adding colour to food or helping to preserve it. Each country has regulations that outline which additives can be used, in what quantity they can be used, and in what type of foods they can be used.

All additives have a name and a number assigned to them. The numbering system for additives in Europe currently has the letter E followed by the number. An international numbering system is being developed and, in the majority of cases, the European numbers correspond to it.

Some additives are restricted to use in a limited number of foods whereas others are allowed at whatever level is necessary to achieve the desired technical effect (this is referred to as "quantum satis") and no limit is set. Some additives have been allocated a figure for acceptable daily intake (ADI) and others have not.

Accessing information within European legislation, with the constant amendments and updates, is like entering an intricate maze without a map. Thankfully, there are initiatives under way to attempt to simplify the way information is presented.

Below you will find a list of the 326 food additives that were allowed in the European Union at the time of writing this second edition.

EU List of Additives

E100 Curcumin

E101 (i) Riboflavin (ii) Riboflavin-5'-phosphate

E102 Tartrazine

E104 Quinoline Yellow

E110 Sunset Yellow FCF, Orange Yellow S

E120 Cochineal, Carminic acid, Carmines

E122 Azorubine, Carmoisine

E123 Amaranth

E124 Ponceau 4R, Cochineal Red A

E127 Erythrosine

E128 Red 2G

E129 Allura Red AC

E131 Patent Blue V

E132 Indigotine, Indigo carmine

E133 Brilliant Blue FCF

E140 Chlorophylis and Chlorophyllins: (i) Chlorophylls (ii) Chlorophyllins

E141 Copper complexes of chlorophylls and chlorophyllins (i) Copper complexes of chlorophylls (ii) Copper complexes of chlorophyllins

E142 Greens S

E150a Plain caramel

E150b Caustic sulphite caramel

E150c Ammonia caramel

E150d Sulphite ammonia caramel

E151 Brilliant Black BN, Black PN

E153 Vegetable carbon

E154 Brown FK

E155 Brown HT

E160a Carotenes: (i) Mixed carotenes (ii) Beta-carotene

E160b Annatto, bixin, norbixin

E160c Paprika extract, capsanthin, capsorubin
E160d Lycopene
E160e Beta-apo-8'-carotenal (C 30)
E160f Ethyl ester of beta-apo-8'-carotenic acid (C 30)
E161b Lutein
E161g Canthaxanthin
E162 Beetroot Red, betanin
E163 Anthocyanins
E170 Calcium carbonates
E171 Titanium dioxide
E172 Iron oxides and hydroxides
E173 Aluminium
E174 Silver
E175 Gold
E180 Latolrubine BK
E200 Sorbic acid
E202 Potassium sorbate
E203 Calcium sorbate
E210 Benzoic acid
E211 Sodium benzoate
E212 Potassium benzoate
E213 Calcium benzoate
E214 Ethyl p-hydroxybenzoate
E215 Sodium ethyl p-hydroxybenzoate
E218 Methyl p-hydroxybenzoate
E219 Sodium methyl p-hydroxybenzoate
E220 Sulphur dioxide
E221 Sodium sulphite
E222 Sodium hydrogen sulphite
E223 Sodium metabisulphite
E224 Potassium metabisulphite
E226 Calcium sulphite
E227 Calcium hydrogen sulphite

E228 Potassium hydrogen sulphite
E230 Biphenyl, diphenyl
E231 Orthophenyl phenol
E232 Sodium orthophenyl phenol
E234 Nisin
E235 Natamycin
E239 Hexamethylene tetramine
E242 Dimethyl dicarbonate
E249 Potassium nitrite
E250 Sodium nitrite
E251 Sodium nitrate
E252 Potassium nitrate
E260 Acetic acid
E261 Potassium acetate
E262 Sodium acetates (i) Sodium acetate (ii) Sodium hydrogen
acetate (sodium diacetate)
E263 Calcium acetate
E270 Lactic acid
E280 Propionic acid
E281 Sodium propionate
E282 Calcium propionate
E283 Potassium propionate
E284 Boric acid
E285 Sodium tetraborate (borax)
E290 Carbon dioxide
E296 Malic acid
E297 Fumaric acid
E300 Ascorbic acid
E301 Sodium ascorbate
E302 Calcium ascorbate
E304 Fatty acid esters of ascorbic acid (i) Ascorbyl palmitate
(ii) Ascorbyl stearate
E306 Tocopherol-rich extract

E307 Alpha-tocopherol

E308 Gamma-tocopherol

E309 Delta-tocopherol

E310 Propyl gallate

E311 Octyl gallate

E312 Dodecyl gallate

E315 Erythorbic acid

E316 Sodium erythorbate

E319 Tertiary-butyl hydroquinone (TBHQ)

E320 Butylated hydroxyanisole (BHA)

E321 Butylated hydroxytoluene (BHT)

E322 Lecithins

E325 Sodium lactate

E326 Potassium lactate

E327 Calcium lactate

E330 Citric acid

E331 Sodium citrates (i) Monosodium citrate (ii) Disodium citrate (iii) Trisodium citrate

E332 Potassium citrates (i) Monopotassium citrate (ii) Tripotassium citrate

E333 Calcium citrates (i) Monocalcium citrate (ii) Dicalcium citrate (iii) Tricalcium citrate

E334 Tartaric acid (L(+)-)

E335 Sodium tartrates (i) Monosodium tartrate (ii) Disodium tartrate

E336 Potassium tartrates (i) Monopotassium tartrate (ii) Dipotassium tartrate

E337 Sodium potassium tartrate

E338 Phosphoric acid

E339 Sodium phosphates (i) Monosodium phosphate (ii) Disodium phosphate (iii) Trisodium phosphate

E340 Potassium phosphates (i) Monopotassium phosphate (ii) Dipotassium phosphate (iii) Tripotassium phosphate

E341 Calcium phosphates (i) Monocalcium phosphate (ii) Dicalcium phosphate (iii) Tricalcium phosphate

E343 Magnesium phosphates (i) monomagnesium phosphate (ii) Dimagnesium phosphate

E350 Sodium malates (i) Sodium malate (ii) Sodium hydrogen malate

E351 Potassium malate

E352 Calcium malates (i) Calcium malate (ii) Calcium hydrogen malate

E353 Metatartaric acid

E354 Calcium tartrate

E355 Adipic acid

E356 Sodium adipate

E357 Potassium adipate

E363 Succinic acid

E380 Triammonium citrate

E385 Calcium disodium ethylene diamine tetra-acetate (Calcium disodium EDTA)

E392 Extracts of rosemary (Extract of rosemary leaf (antioxidant))

E400 Alginic acid

E401 Sodium alginate

E402 Potassium alginate

E403 Ammonium alginate

E404 Calcium alginate

E405 Propan-1,2-diol alginate

E406 Agar

E407 Carrageenan

E407a Processed eucheuma seaweed

E410 Locust bean gum

E412 Guar gum

E413 Tragacanth

E414 Acacia gum (gum arabic)

E415 Xanthan gum

E416 Karaya gum

E417 Tara gum

E418 Gellan gum

E420 Sorbitol (i) Sorbitol (ii) Sorbitol syrup

E421 Mannitol

E422 Glycerol

E425 Konjac (i) Konjac gum (ii) Konjac glucomannane

E426 Soybean hemicellulose

E427 Cassia gum

E431 Polyoxyethylene (40) stearate

E432 Polyoxyethylene sorbitan monolaurate (polysorbate 20)

E433 Polyoxyethylene sorbitan monooleate (polysorbate 80)

E434 Polyoxyethylene sorbitan monopalmitate (polysorbate 40)

E435 Polyoxyethylene sorbitan monostearate (polysorbate 60)

E436 Polyoxyethylene sorbitan tristearate (polysorbate 65)

E440 Pectins (i) pectin (ii) amidated pectin

E442 Ammonium phosphatides

E444 Sucrose acetate isobutyrate

E445 Glycerol esters of wood rosins

E450 Diphosphates: (i) Disodium diphosphate (Disodium dihydrogen diphosphate, Disodium dihydrogen pyrophosphate, Sodium acid pyrophosphate, Disodium pyrophosphate); (ii) Trisodium diphosphate (Acid trisodium pyrophosphate, Trisodium monohydrogen diphosphate); (iii) Tetrasodium diphosphate (Tetrasodium pyrophosphate, Sodium pyrophosphate); (iv) Dipotassium diphosphate (v) Tetrapotassium diphosphate (Potassium pyrophosphate, Tetrapotassium pyrophosphate); (vi) Dicalcium diphosphate (Calcium pyrophosphate); (vii) Calcium dihydrogen diphosphate (Acid calcium pyrophosphate, Monocalcium dihydrogen pyrophosphate)

E451 Triphosphates: (i) Pentasodium triphosphate (pentasodium tripolyphosphate, sodium tripolyphosphate); (ii) Pentapotassium triphosphate (Pentapotassium tripolyphosphate, Potassium triphosphate, Potassium tripolyphosphate)

E452 Polyphosphates: (i) Sodium polyphosphates (Sodium hexametaphosphate, Sodium tetrapolyphosphate, Graham's salt, Sodium polyphosphates, glassy, Sodium polymetaphosphate, Sodium metaphosphate, Insoluble sodium metaphosphate, Maddrell's salt, Insoluble sodium polyphosphate, IMP); (ii) Potassium polyphosphates (Potassium metaphosphate, Potassium polymetaphosphate, Kurrol salt); (iii) Sodium calcium polyphosphate (Sodium calcium polyphosphate, glassy); (iv) Calcium polyphophates (Calcium metaphosphate, Calcium polymetaphosphate)

E459 Beta-cyclodextrine

E460 Cellulose (i) Microcrystalline cellulose (ii) Powdered cellulose

E461 Methyl cellulose

E462 Ethyl cellulose

E463 Hydroxypropyl cellulose

E464 Hydroxypropyl methyl cellulose

E465 Ethyl methyl cellulose

E466 Carboxy methyl cellulose, Sodium carboxy methyl cellulose

E468 Crosslinked sodium carboxymethyl cellulose

E469 Enzymically hydrolysed carboxy methyl cellulose

E470a Sodium, potassium and calcium salts of fatty acids

E470b Magnesium salts of fatty acids

E471 Mono- and diglycerides of fatty acids

E472a Acetic acid esters of mono- and diglycerides of fatty acids

E472b Lactic acid esters of mono- and diglycerides of fatty acids

E472c Citric acid esters of mono- and diglycerides of fatty acids

E472d Tartaric acid esters of mono- and diglycerides of fatty acids

E472e Mono- and diacetyl tartaric acid esters of mono- and diglycerides of fatty acids

E472f Mixed acetic and tartaric acid esters of mono- and diglycerides of fatty acids

E473 Sucrose esters of fatty acids

E474 Sucroglycerides

E475 Polyglycerol esters of fatty acids

E476 Polyglycerol polyricinoleate

E477 Propane-1,2-diol esters of fatty acids

E479b Thermally oxidized soya bean oil interacted with mono- and diglycerides of fatty acids

E481 Sodium stearoyl-2-lactylate

E482 Calcium stearoyl-2-lactylate

E483 Stearyl tartrate

E491 Sorbitan monostearate

E492 Sorbitan tristearate

E493 Sorbitan monolaurate

E494 Sorbitan monooleate

E495 Sorbitan monopalmitate

E500 Sodium carbonates (i) Sodium carbonate (ii) Sodium hydrogen carbonate (iii) Sodium sesquicarbonate

E501 Potassium carbonates (i) Potassium carbonate (ii) Potassium hydrogen carbonate

E503 Ammonium carbonates (i) Ammonium carbonate (ii) Ammonium hydrogen carbonate E504 Magnesium carbonates (i) Magnesium carbonate (ii) Magnesium hydroxide carbonate (syn. Magnesium hydrogen carbonate)

E507 Hydrochloric acid

E508 Potassium chloride

E509 Calcium chloride

E511 Magnesium chloride

E512 Stannous chloride

E513 Sulphuric acid

E514 Sodium sulphates (i) Sodium sulphate (ii) Sodium hydrogen sulphate

E515 Potassium sulphates (i) Potassium sulphate (ii) Potassium hydrogen sulphate E516 Calcium sulphate

E517 Ammonium sulphate

E520 Aluminium sulphate

E521 Aluminium sodium sulphate

E522 Aluminium potassium sulphate

E523 Aluminium ammonium sulphate

E524 Sodium hydroxide

E525 Potassium hydroxide

E526 Calcium hydroxide

E527 Ammonium hydroxide

E528 Magnesium hydroxide

E529 Calcium oxide

E530 Magnesium oxide

E535 Sodium ferrocyanide

E536 Potassium ferrocyanide

E538 Calcium ferrocyanide

E541 Sodium aluminium phosphate, acidic

E551 Silicon dioxide

E552 Calcium silicate

E553a (i) Magnesium silicate (ii) Magnesium trisilicate

E553b Talc
E554 Sodium aluminium silicate
E555 Potassium aluminium silicate
E556 Calcium aluminium silicate
E558 Bentonite
E559 Aluminium silicate (Kaolin)
E570 Fatty acids
E574 Gluconic acid
E575 Glucono-delta-lactone
E576 Sodium gluconate
E577 Potassium gluconate
E578 Calcium gluconate
E579 Ferrous gluconate
E585 Ferrous lactate
E586 4-hexylresorcinol
E620 Glutamic acid
E621 Monosodium glutamate
E622 Monopotassium glutamate
E623 Calcium diglutamate
E624 Monoammonium glutamate
E625 Magnesium diglutamate
E626 Guanylic acid
E627 Disodium guanylate
E628 Dipotassium guanylate
E629 Calcium guanylate
E630 Inosinic acid
E631 Disodium inosinate
E632 Dipotassium inosinate
E633 Calcium inosinate
E634 Calcium 5'-ribonucleotides
E635 Disodium 5'-ribonucleotides
E640 Glycine and its sodium salt
E650 Zinc acetate

E900 Dimethyl polysiloxane
E901 Beeswax, white and yellow
E902 Candelillla wax
E903 Carnauba wax
E904 Shellac
E905 Microcrystalline wax
E907 Hydrogenated poly-1-decene
E912 Montanic acid esters
E914 Oxidized polyethylene wax
E920 L-Cysteine
E927b Carbamide
E938 Argon
E939 Helium
E941 Nitrogen
E942 Nitrous oxide
E943a Butane
E943b Isobutane
E944 Propane
E948 Oxygen
E949 Hydrogen
E950 Acesulfame K
E951 Aspartame
E952 Cyclamic acid and its Na and Ca salts
E953 Isomalt
E954 Saccharin and its Na, K and Ca salts
E955 Sucralose
E957 Thaumatin
E959 NeohesperidineDC
E 961 Neotame
E962 Salt of aspartame - acesulfame
E965 Maltitol (i) Maltitol (ii) Maltitol syrup
E966 Lactitol
E967 Xylitol

E968 Erythritol
E999 Quilllaia extract
E1103 Invertase
E1105 Lysozyme
E1200 Polydextrose
E1201 Polyvinylpyrrolidone
E1202 Polyvinylpolypyrrolidone
E1203 Polyvinyl alcohol (Vinyl alcohol polymer, PVOH)
E1204 Pullulan
E1404 Oxidized starch
E1410 Monostarch phosphate
E1412 Distarch phosphate
E1413 Phosphated distarch phosphate
E1414 Acetylated distarch phosphate
E1420 Acetylated starch
E1422 Acetylated distarch adipate
E1440 Hydroxy propyl starch
E1442 Hydroxy propyl distarch phosphate
E1450 Starch sodium octenyl succinate
E1451 Acetylated oxidised starch
E1452 Starch aluminium octenyl succinate
E1505 Triethyl citrate
E1517 Glyceryl diacetate (diacetin)
E1518 Glyceryl triacetate (triacetin)
E1519 Benzyl alcohol
E1520 Propan-1,2-diol (propylene glycol)
E1521 Polyethylene glycols (PEG, Macrogol, Polyethylene oxide)

Resources

Information on the International Standard can be found on the Codex Alimentarius site:
http://www.codexalimentarius.org/

Information on the European regulations can be accessed via the EU site:
http://ec.europa.eu/

Information specific to individual countries can be found via that country's government website. In the UK information can be obtained via the Food Standards Agency (http://www.food.gov.uk/) or the main government site (http://www.direct.gov.uk)

If you keep a detailed food diary and have any concerns about a particular additive you will be able to find out more about the additive by searching on line. General searches may provide the information you are seeking but if they don't then try searching through research papers at a site such as PubMed (http://www.ncbi.nlm.nih.gov/pubmed/).

Index